THE STORY
OF BIOETHICS

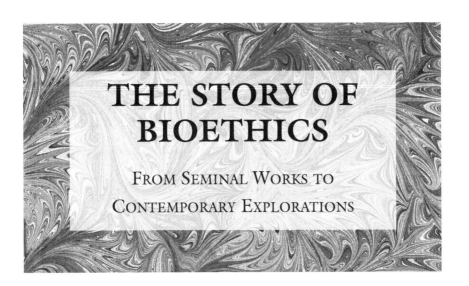

THE STORY OF BIOETHICS

FROM SEMINAL WORKS TO CONTEMPORARY EXPLORATIONS

JENNIFER K. WALTER

Eran P. Klein

EDITORS

GEORGETOWN UNIVERSITY PRESS
Washington, D.C.

Georgetown University Press, Washington, D.C.
© 2003 by Georgetown University Press. All rights reserved.
Printed in the United States of America

10 9 8 7 6 5 4 3 2 1   2003

This book is printed on acid-free recycled paper meeting the requirements
of the American National Standard for Permanence in Paper for Printed
Library Materials.

Library of Congress Cataloging-in-Publication Data

The story of bioethics : from seminal works to contemporary explorations /
Jennifer K. Walter and Eran P. Klein, editors.
        p. cm.
Includes bibliographical references and index.
    ISBN 0-87840-138-5 (pbk. : alk. paper)
1. Bioethics—History. I. Walter, Jennifer K. (Jennifer Kay), 1976–
II. Klein, Eran P. (Eran Patrick)
    QH332.S77   2003
    174′.957—dc21

                                                        2003004678

To all those who have taught us,

in varying capacities, about medicine,

philosophy, and the important things in life.

CONTENTS

Part Three: Boundaries and Issues of
Inclusion in Bioethics

ERAN P. KLEIN AND JENNIFER K. WALTER

If critical self-reflection is a mark of maturity, bioethics as a field seems to be coming of age. As Albert R. Jonsen notes in his recent history, bioethics—while not emerging de novo—was only "born" as a distinct discipline over the last several decades (Jonsen 1998). Set against the long history of philosophy and theology proper (out of which, arguably, bioethics arose), bioethics as a field is indeed young. Yet the diversity and depth of ideas that have emerged during its short lifetime are impressive. The rapid social changes wrought by modern medicine have required that bioethics be precocious beyond its years. Unlike fields with longer histories, the accelerated development of bioethics has left little time for reflection on the shape of the field itself. This is beginning to change.

In recent years, interest in bioethics as a field has largely come from two directions. The first has been a historical interest in the origins of bioethics—the events, people, social movements, and technological advancements present at the start of the field. The second has been an interest in the purpose and potential of bioethics as a field—what role can or should national commissions play? What are bioethics programs training people for? Are there bioethics "experts"? How diverse is bioethics in terms of race, class, religion, and ideology? Put simply, there are two questions that motivate interest in bioethics as a field: From where did bioethics come and where is it going?

The essays collected in this volume are premised on the notion that these two threads are interwoven: one cannot understand where bioethics is going as a field without understanding how it arrived where it is today, nor can one talk intelligibly about the history of bioethics without a sense of how it understands itself today and projects itself into the future. This volume finds seminal works in bioethics to be a particularly useful resource for exploring the connection between the past and future of the field. Insofar as seminal works have had a role in establishing the field of bioethics, they have historical importance. Insofar as they continue to shape the nature and scope of debate in contemporary bioethics, they are inextricably bound with its future. Seminal works provide a unique window into understanding the field of bioethics.

There are certain features of bioethics that make an examination of the field's seminal works especially valuable. First, the role that seminal works play in bioethics seems different from the roles that seminal works play in both the sciences and the humanities. This would seem to be a consequence of the unique position that bioethics maintains between the sciences and the humanities. Second, the accelerated development of bioethics has required that many of its seminal works be *works in transition*. Third, given that bioethics is an interdisciplinary field comprising theology, philosophy, sociology, and so on, seminal works have to be *bridging works* in that they develop out of the current discussions in these fields and must speak to their individual and overlapping concerns.

The natural sciences and the humanities accord different roles to their seminal works. In the sciences, these works tend to possess more historical than pedagogical value. Few biologists read the original Mendel, few physicists Newton, and few chemists Lavoisier. The sciences generally are oriented toward solving problems of today and tomorrow. Interest in seminal works in the natural sciences tends to be reserved for those with a penchant for the history of a particular field or idea, not for those actively engaged in scientific pursuit. In the humanities, on the other hand, seminal works tend to carry more than historical value. Students of philosophy or theology are encouraged to read the original Kant or Aquinas. Seminal works tend to be the starting point of pedagogy in these fields.

Bioethics is a field that finds its home somewhere between the humanities and the natural sciences, and the role it accords its seminal works reflects this. Like the natural sciences, bioethics tends to orient itself toward the future. What bioethical issues lie on the horizon? What can be done about them *now*? Few bioethicists go back and read the transcripts of the Nuremberg trials or the final report of the National Commission for the Protection of Human Subjects of Biomedical and Behavioral Research. Typically only those with a quite narrow or historical interest do so. Yet bioethics does call on seminal works in certain important ways. Like the humanities, bioethics values argument and diversity of views and tends to be somewhat skeptical of consensus. Seminal works are frequently appealed to in order to motivate discussion or contrary lines of argument (see for example Judith Jarvis Thomson's famous article on abortion: Thomson 1971). The unique role that seminal works play in bioethics is in large part a function of the relationship of bioethics to the humanities and the natural sciences.

The rapid development of bioethics as a field has required that works in bioethics often be taken as works in transition. The ongoing changes in medical technology and the exigencies of medical practice make this necessary. Works are published and ideas elucidated in the absence of a settled empirical base. As a result, works in bioethics are often understood (as James Childress notes in this volume) as "works in progress," with an implicit understanding that new empirical developments will likely require that concepts be adjusted, refined, or further elucidated. The most obvious evidence of this is the elevated importance of revised works in bioethics (e.g., Beauchamp and Childress's *Principles of Biomedical Ethics*). That bioethics is a field built upon works in transition does not mean that it lacks a canon. Rather it has a canon in a unique way. It may be true that few in bioethics have read all the editions of Beauchamp and Childress's *Principles of Biomedical Ethics*, yet nearly everyone versed in the field has read or been influenced by this work. The canon of bioethics is comprised largely of works in transition.

Bioethics is an interdisciplinary field and its seminal works reflect this as well. As LeRoy Walters discusses in the afterword to this volume, from its earliest years the field has welcomed diverse religious and disciplinary voices. This has meant that works in bioethics have often crossed over traditional boundaries. Such works have been written to speak not only to individuals from different traditions within a single discipline (e.g., philosophical consequentialists and deontologists) but to individuals from different religious backgrounds (e.g., Protestants and Catholics) and cultural upbringings (e.g., Western and Eastern). Several of the works discussed in this volume (Beauchamp and Childress's *Principles of Biomedical Ethics*, Curran's *Politics, Medicine, and Christian Ethics: A Dialogue with Paul Ramsey*, and Reich's two editions of the *Encyclopedia of Bioethics*) are paradigmatic examples of the bridging character of works in bioethics.

This volume assembles a diverse group of specialists who are at the top of their own fields and have also been recognized as having contributed seminal works in the field of bioethics. In our discussions with leaders in the field, we selected books, encyclopedias, and commissions that have had the most staying power, albeit through several editions, and have provided the lens through which the field continues to be examined. To make our task more manageable, and in honor of the thirtieth anniversary of the Kennedy Institute of Ethics, we limited our selection of scholars to those who had been associated with the Kennedy Institute in its early years. Consequently, we in no way claim to have produced a comprehensive list of the seminal works in bioethics. Instead, we take ourselves to have identified an important subset of these works.

Each chapter in this volume has three distinct sections. The first is the work's historical context both from the vantage point of the author's own intellectual history and from his or her view of the state of the field at the time of publication. The second section is a conceptual overview of the work, which summarizes some of the main themes and provides the reader an opportunity to contrast the different views presented in different chapters. Finally, the third section is the work's current relevance (i.e., how the work fits into current debates). Authors address different aspects of current relevance by engaging in discussions with their contemporaries and fielding continuing criticisms of their views, by taking on current bioethical issues and demonstrating how their original views can be adapted to accommodate developing concerns, and by providing suggestions about where the field as a whole needs to continue to expand and pursue greater depth of focus.

The book is divided into three sections. In the first, the question of theory in bioethics is addressed. Edmund D. Pellegrino offers an approach to theory in bioethics that takes as its starting point the essentially normative character of medical practice. Tom L. Beauchamp and James F. Childress each give their own take on the proper role of principles in bioethics, and discuss which criticisms of their appeal to principles over the years have been most trenchant. Robert M. Veatch provides an updated and concise formulation of a contractual approach to theory in medical ethics. And H. Tristram Engelhardt, Jr., in typical fashion, gives an eloquent and biting critique of traditional accounts of theory in bioethics before suggesting what he takes to be his more modest view of the subject. These chapters on theory in bioethics contain modifications, enhancements, or elucidations of the original theories presented in the seminal works of these authors and represent the accommodation, in some cases, of their colleagues' views. In keeping with the dialogue between these authors that has occurred publicly throughout the years, many of the chapters advance the debate by more clearly delineating the points of similarity and conflict between the different theories.

The second section takes up the question of what role theology, given the religious roots of bioethics, can play in the *future* of the field. Charles E. Curran explains why Catholic moral theology became so involved in bioethics at the creation of the field and traces its heritage into the modern day and the future. The depth of analysis that moral theology has brought to bioethics is demonstrated in Lisa Sowle Cahill's reminiscences on

Richard A. McCormick's work. Protestant theologian William F. May employs traditionally religious language of covenant as a means for understanding the physician's role in modern medicine.

The final section of the book addresses questions about the shape and inclusiveness of the field of bioethics. Writing on the evolution of the *Encyclopedia of Bioethics,* Warren T. Reich is specifically concerned with how the boundaries of the field of bioethics are drawn. He is concerned not only with which disciplines and theoretical approaches are given voice in bioethics, but also with what countries, which patients, which class, race, and gender should be given emphasis in the field. In her discussion of research on vulnerable groups, Patricia A. King discusses the challenges and potential hurdles in achieving just and nonabusive inclusion in medical research. The book concludes with LeRoy Walters' essay on the founding and evolution of the Kennedy Institute of Ethics.

REFERENCES

Jonsen, Albert. 1998. *The Birth of Bioethics.* New York: Oxford University Press.

Thomson, Judith Jarvis. 1971. A Defense of Abortion. *Philosophy and Public Affairs* 1, no. 1: 47–66.

ACKNOWLEDGMENTS

This volume developed out of a conference held at Georgetown University in honor of the thirtieth anniversary of the Kennedy Institute of Ethics. The conference, and hence this book, would not have been possible without financial and other support from a number of individuals, departments, and schools at Georgetown University, including then Provost Dorothy Brown and the Office of the Provost, Dean Jane D. McAuliffe and Georgetown College, Wayne Davis and the Department of Philosophy, Dean Judith Areen and the Georgetown University Law Center, Dean Stephen Ray Mitchell and the Georgetown Medical Center's Medical Student Parents' Council, and most importantly, Madison Powers and the Kennedy Institute of Ethics. The support provided by Madison and the administrative burden shared by Linda Powell and Sally Schofield were instrumental to the success of the conference. We would also like to thank the respondents to the original papers presented at the conference: John Collins Harvey, M.D., Ph.D.; Kevin Wm. Wildes, S.J., Ph.D.; Carol M. Spicer, Ph.D.; Francis Kane, Ph.D.; David D. DeGrazia, Ph.D.; Margaret Little, Ph.D.; James J. Walter, Ph.D.; Jeffrey Kahn, Ph.D.; John P. Langan, S.J., Ph.D.; and Daniel Sulmasy, O.F.M., M.D., Ph.D. for engaging the participants in dialogue and challenging them in insightful ways.

We would like to extend our utmost gratitude to both John P. Langan and James J. Walter for serving as patient and thoughtful advisers throughout every aspect of the conception and execution of this volume. Additionally, we would like to acknowledge the many contributors to this volume who shared their expertise and patience with their novice editors. We hope this book stands as a concrete sign of the faith these contributors and Georgetown University Press's director Richard Brown placed in two bioethics graduate students. We would also like to acknowledge the Graduate Biomedical Committee, the Georgetown Medical School, and the Philosophy Department for supporting the M.D./Ph.D. in bioethics program at Georgetown.

Finally, we would like to acknowledge the continued and unfaltering support of our families and friends. Your continued interest in our finishing this volume has made it possible and your continued interest in us has made it enjoyable. Eran would particularly like to thank Nilana Gunasekaran.

PART ONE
THEORIES IN BIOETHICS

From Medical Ethics to a Moral Philosophy of the Professions

EDMUND D. PELLEGRINO

When I joined the Kennedy Institute of Ethics in 1978, I was no stranger to medical ethics. I had been reading and studying the subject since 1940, my junior year in college. My major field of study was chemistry. However, pre–World War I Catholic colleges required four years of philosophy and four of theology regardless of what undergraduate major field one chose to study. I was fortunate in that these subjects were just as fascinating to me as chemistry. As a result, both fields provided the launching pad for my later scholarly research in the laboratory and in philosophy.

I was first introduced to medical ethics by my college professors, who lent me books and papers in medical ethics taken from the 400-year-old Roman Catholic tradition of medical morality. I was thus sensitized to the indispensability of medical ethics to the practice of medicine and to my personal integrity as a Roman Catholic physician. I read and discussed the issues then current without the slightest doubt about their relevance to my future medical practice. At that time, Aldous Huxley's *Brave New World*, published in 1932, had already provided arresting insights into the complex ethical and social issues that could result from progress in human and animal biology. Debates about genetics, artificial placentas, biotechnology, and technocracy were already under way in class and in conversations outside class. Earlier "sci-fi" novels by Jules Verne and H. G. Wells foresaw the technological possibilities of time and space travel. George Orwell's *1984*, published later in 1949, gave a graphic and chilling picture of a technocratic society. The "brave new world" was already a visible ethical morass, and the need for ethical constraints on the advance of technology was appreciated.

These imaginative literary prognostications were not evident in medical practice when I entered medical school. In 1941, specific treatments that effectively changed the natural history of disease were scant in number. The list was a small one: arsenic for syphilis, liver extract for "pernicious anemia," quinine for malaria, insulin for diabetes, digitalis for heart failure, and a few others. Medicine's dramatic and unprecedented power to alter the human condition was still a promissory note.

To be sure, the sulfonamides had made their appearance a few years earlier. Penicillin came to us in my final year in school as a dirty colored powder in a vial to be used experimentally to treat pneumonia and subacute bacterial endocarditis. This was the beginning of the era, prematurely dubbed the "conquest of infectious disease." The basic science and the pharmacological and genetic intricacies of today's medicine were scarcely imagined. Medical ethics in consequence was largely confined to professional ethics, taught, if at all, as a set of precepts to be followed, not a subject for critical ethical appraisal.

In my own case, I do not recall medical ethics being mentioned, except in small informal discussions among students and residents. Catholic students did worry about certain dilemmas associated with obstetrical practice. For the most part it was assumed that we would discover what was right on our own. Among both Catholics and non-Catholics abortion and euthanasia were almost universally condemned, as were the "corporate practice" of medicine and for-profit doctor-owned hospitals.

Some passing references to the traditions of medical ethics were made in discussions in a medical history club. But since my class was on an accelerated schedule, finishing the whole curriculum in three years because of World War II, there was really no time for reflective thinking. My own reading continued, however, through my medical school residency years.

I myself began to teach medical ethics at the bedside to residents and medical students in 1960 when I became chairman of the department of medicine at the University of Kentucky. I first began then to write and publish on a variety of topics in medical ethics and the humanities in medicine (McElhinney and Pellegrino 2001, 291–317). I approached these topics then, as I do now, from an Aristotelian-Thomist realist stance and with a scholastic taste for distinctions and definitions.

In the mid-1960s, it became clear that most of medical ethics was really medical morality—a set of assertions and moral precepts without a formal groundwork of ethical justification or argumentation. While many of these moral precepts might be valid, without a justifiable ethical foundation they could easily be challenged, denied, or compromised. This is indeed what happened when medical morals were subjected to critical philosophical inquiry in the early 1970s.

Professional philosophers began to take medical ethics seriously and to look for principled arguments for the resolution of professional and clinical ethical dilemmas. This was a departure, since until that time philosophers had largely ignored medical ethics. Even physician-philosophers like John Locke, Karl Jaspers, or William James failed to do a systemic analysis of the ethics of their original professions. To be sure, Plato, Aristotle, and the Stoics used medicine to illustrate their philosophical arguments. But none produced a treatise on medical ethics itself (Jaspers 1963).

When serious study of medical ethics was initiated, it consisted largely in the application of existing philosophical or theological systems to medicine. These systems were "applied" or, better, superimposed on medicine and its practice. None derived an ethic of medicine beginning with medicine or looking at the nature of medicine itself as a special kind of human activity.

At the same time, historical and sociological critics disassembled the Hippocratic ethic and ethos. The ancient idea of a universal set of duties binding all physicians as physicians across time and national boundaries was seriously eroded. Demands for a "new" ethic more suitable to the times and mores multiplied and continue to this day. The whole enterprise of medical and professional ethics was headed to definition by social convention and consensus, a pathway I believed then and believe now to be deleterious to patients and to society.

Contravening these trends, I thought then, and I think now, that the ethics of medicine should be based in the nature of the medical relationship, that is, in a philosophy *of* medicine. My thesis then was, and remains, that the obligations specific to physicians arise from the special features of the personal relationship between the person who is ill and the person the ill person seeks for help. The resulting relationship has certain features that give it a special character that generates special mutual moral duties.

This does not mean that medical ethics is isolated from general ethics or that the principles, rules, and duties of medical ethics as a discipline are self-justifying. It does, I believe, mean that the determination of which principles, duties, and virtues are most pertinent is linked to the nature of the human relationships that are central to the clinical encounter. The exploration of the existential, experiential, and phenomenological aspects of being ill, professing to heal, and healing seemed the most likely starting point for a philosophy of medicine and the first step to the ethics of medicine.

This approach fitted well with my own years of expertise as a clinician and with my earlier training in the realism of existential Thomism and some of its extensions in phenomenological realism (Von Hildebrand 1973; Seifert 1984). I had been introduced to the possibilities of the phenomenological method through my friendship and conversations with Professor Erwin Straus. I did not accept the transcendental dimensions of Husserl's philosophy but Straus helped me to see in his critique of the Cartesianism of modern psychology that the primacy of the world of the senses could be recovered (Straus 1963).

Indeed, my contact with Professor Straus led me to my first effort to link philosophy and medicine (Pellegrino 1966, 272–84). This was my first effort at a philosophy of medicine in its broadest terms. It revealed my conviction that a philosophical anthropology was an existential element in any moral philosophy for medicine. It was also behind my interest in developing a journal linking philosophy and medicine. These ideas were further developed by others and by me in the early issues of the *Journal of Medicine and Philosophy*, which was first published in 1976.

In 1976 I published my own first attempt to ground an ethic of medicine in a specific philosophy of medicine, that is, in a philosophy of the interpersonal relationship between physician and patient in the "clinical encounter"—that moment when a decision and action must be taken which will be for the good of the patient, both technically and morally (Pellegrino 1976, 35–56). In that paper I argued that three phenomena of the clinical encounter should serve as the starting point of a definition of what makes medicine what it is. This paper later served as the starting point for *A Philosophical Basis of Medical Practice* (Pellegrino and Thomasma 1981), and in fact an extended version of it forms the first chapter of that work.

These three phenomena were (1) the existential fact of illness or disease, (2) the act of promise or profession by the physician who offers to help the patient caught in the predicament of illness, and (3) the act of medicine—making the technically right and the morally good decision that best serves the needs of the sick person as grasped by that person and her physician. The close relationship of these three universal phenomena—being ill, promising to heal, and healing itself—provided a foundation in the real world for the obligations of the physician and patient to each other.

I argued that illness wounded our humanity, challenged our self-image, limited our freedom in special ways, and made us vulnerable ontologically and existentially. A physician who offered to help a human in this altered existential state incurred obligations to act in such a way that the purpose of the encounter—healing, helping, caring, curing—could be achieved. The primacy of the good of the patient was the *locus ethicus* of the relationship. This primacy could only be preserved if physicians are competent, discern the complex nature of the patient's good, are compassionate, practice some degree of suppression of self-interest, and protect the inherent dignity of the patient as a human person.

On this view, the immediate telos of the clinical relationship is the good of the patient or, in more clinical terms, a right and good healing and helping act. If this telos or end is to be achieved, certain character traits are entailed—fidelity, trust, benevolence, truth telling, intellectual honesty, humility, courage, suppression of self-interest—at a minimum. These character traits are entailed not because they are admirable; they are admirable because they are essential to achieving the ends and purposes of medicine. These ends derive from the realities of the clinical encounter and not from societal convention, construction, negotiated agreement, or contract.

Many of these duties and virtues were expressed or implied in the Hippocratic oath and the deontological books of the corpus. But they do not derive their moral authority because they are in the oath. The oath simply reflects the moral content of the patient-physician personal healing and helping relationship (Pellegrino 2001, 70–87). My hope has been that my analysis of the source of the doctor's obligations and virtues will give moral substance to the oath and explain why it has had such a long-standing place of influence in medical ethics.

I do not assert that medical ethics is the privileged domain of the doctor, but that it is imposed on the doctor by the very nature of what he purports to do as a physician. Nor do I argue that medicine is the only healing profession defined by these moral considerations. Indeed, as my subsequent work, alone and with David Thomasma, emphasizes, they are requisite features of the other health professions and of other professions. Each helping profession confronts vulnerable, dependent, and anxious human beings and possesses and professes the special knowledge and skill needed by those persons.

I also hold that these realities of the clinical encounter reflect universal human needs experienced by human beings in whatever era, cultural milieu, or ethnic category they exist. They are in fact human experiences modified by culture and history but not in any essential way. These were the realities that faced the Hippocratic physicians, the Shaman, medicine man, or curandero, as well as the technologically trained physician of today and tomorrow. As long as humans are mortal, become ill, and are altered existentially by illness and disease, they will need help, healing, caring, and curing. The relationship may be mediated and modulated by culture, technology, or spiritual belief, but its fundamental human grounding will not disappear.

Thomasma and I developed these themes in a series of books. In the first, *A Philosophical Basis of Medical Practice*, we developed our most fundamental statement of the philosophical basis of medical practice, which we grounded in a philosophy of the body and mind phenomenologically considered (Pellegrino and Thomasma 1981). In a series of books that followed, we explored different dimensions of the vision laid out in *A Philosophical Basis of Medical Practice*. We focused on the complex nature of the patient's good as the telos of the clinical encounter (Pellegrino and Thomasma 1987). This led us to a study of the virtues required of the physician if the telos of the relationship—the good of the patient—was to be attained (Pellegrino and Thomasma 1993). To this we added an analysis of the spiritual virtues entailed by the fact that some physicians also claimed to be Christian (Pellegrino and Thomasma 1996). Our last book went further into the spiritual and religious dimensions of healing and helping (Pellegrino and Thomasma 1997).

As I was preparing this chapter, my friend and coauthor David Thomasma died suddenly and unexpectedly. At the time of his death we were close to the completion of a second edition of our *Philosophical Basis*. I hope I shall be able to complete the task in a way David would have approved. I will sorely miss my collaborator with whom I have worked and from whom I have profited immensely for a quarter of a century.

I cannot do justice to David Thomasma in this essay. So close was our collaboration that it is difficult for me to know who was responsible for any idea, theme, or argument. I can honestly say that in all the time we worked together we never had a falling out of any kind. This I attribute to David's equitable temper, charity, and sense of humor. I will miss his creative mind, his knowledge of the literature, his skill in dissecting my bad ideas, and his generosity with my failings.

As we argued at the beginning of *A Philosophical Basis of Medical Practice*, we took ourselves to be elucidating a philosophy *of* medicine, which we distinguished from philosophy *and* medicine and philosophy *in* medicine. In *A Philosophical Basis of Medical Practice* and in our other individual and independent writings, we have emphasized different aspects of the philosophy of medicine, but on the basic perceptions we were in agreement. Some of our critics have taken us to task for concentrating too much on individual patients, neglecting preventive and social medicine, and for overuse of the "medical model."

We never intended to exclude such considerations. Our aim was to proceed stepwise to develop a paradigm, a philosophy of medicine that could be applied analogically to social medicine, preventive medicine, and to the healing relationships characteristic of the other health professions as well. In the coming second edition of *A Philosophical Basis for Medical Practice*, we address these issues as well as the criticism that we commit the naturalist fallacy.

We have already addressed some of these perceived omissions in separate papers authored collaboratively or individually. As we expanded our notion of a philosophy of medicine, it became clear that we were really developing an existentially grounded philosophy of healing and helping of humans in a state of vulnerability. It has become increasingly apparent too that our philosophy of medicine was also based in a particular notion of the idea of man, that is, a philosophical anthropology and a metaphysical notion of human and social good. Thus we entered the more foundational realm of moral philosophy beyond simply medicine or health care ethics.

We have expanded our consideration beyond medical ethics going progressively from a philosophy of medicine to a philosophy of healing to a philosophy of the health professions. This approach also suggested a way to define a philosophical basis and moral philosophy for other "helping" professions, e.g., law, ministry, teaching. These professions deal, as medicine does, with vulnerable persons: persons in need of justice, learning, or spiritual healing. Law, teaching, and ministry, like medicine, are based in certain empirical phenomena inherent in specific interhuman relationships that entail a moral relationship between the vulnerable and those who serve them.

Let me close with an attempt to relate my own work to the current state of bioethics.[1] Recently, I have continued to explore the basis of a moral philosophy of the health professions and of the professions of law, ministry, and teaching (Pellegrino 2002a, 556–79). Neither this essay nor any of the others is meant to impose what is pejoratively called the "medical model" on other professions. Rather it suggests that there is a phenomenological and real-world similarity in the human existential realities of persons rendered vulnerable by illness, or by a need for justice, spiritual consolation, or knowledge. These phenomena by their nature entail duties, obligations, and virtues of physicians, lawyers, teachers, and ministers. They help to develop a more extended and more credible moral philosophy for the professions more generally than the current sociological interpretations that now prevail.

Let me point out in response to some of my critics that what we have done thus far is not a *compleat* philosophy and ethic of even medicine or health care. We need a fuller explication of the societal dimensions of medicine and its relationships with other professions and society and with preventative medicine. These questions can be approached by a realist examination of the phenomena of the personal and community relationships specific to each of these ways medicine can be manifested. Some of this will be adumbrated in the coming revision of *A Philosophical Basis for Medical Practice*, other parts in a planned work on the social ethics of medicine.

There are a number of interactions and dissonances between the philosophy of medicine and health care that I have espoused from the publication of *A Philosophical Basis of Medical Practice* through to the present, and what I take to be the dominant themes of contemporary bioethics.

First, my view runs contrary to the postmodern insistence on the fallacy of all foundations or overarching ideas in philosophy. It also is "premodern" in its belief in the capacity of reason, albeit limited, to arrive at objective moral truth. The current infatuation with praxis—with what works—is no solid source for either the normative or the morally true.

I do not think a comprehensive moral philosophy, whether in medicine or more generally, is possible without an account of religious and theological sources of moral authority. In the end, faith and reason compliment each other. The ground between them is not an intellectual or conceptual no man's land. There are signs of some lessening in the conflict between them, at least among those ethicists who are not willing entirely to foreclose reflection on these two dimensions of the human spirit. Postmodernists who have sought consolation in moral skepticism have no other place to go. Theologians who scorn reason are similarly constrained. As a result, both are beginning to realize that the boundary between them is not impermeable.

The same can be said of the necessity for a philosophical anthropology. Medicine being simultaneously the scientific and humanistic study of man cannot escape being based in an explicit or implicit philosophy of human nature. Even the denial of such a thing as the "nature" of man, and even those who see only his biological nature, are by these assertions holding a philosophical anthropology.

The genome project, the prospects of human cloning, and the fabrication of human-animal or human-machine hybrids force the question of what it is to be human upon us. When all is said and done the Psalmist's question "What is man?" cannot be evaded (Psalm 8). Clearly the articulation of a philosophy of man and a philosophy of medicine are essential elements in a normative moral philosophy. In this inquiry the philosophy of medicine—of man being ill, suffering, and being healed—fills a place in the complex mosaic of what it means to be human.

My realism and search for objective foundations contravenes the current bioethical trend toward social convention, social construction, and dialogue as means of arriving at transient moral truths. These are valid as methods of political democracy but dangerous. Society is not per se the final arbiter of moral truth. There are sadly too many pathological societies past and present to entrust the canons of morality entirely to politics or social convention. Ethics is not a matter of polls or plebiscites.

My methodological approach is that of Aristotelian-Thomist natural law ethics. While still unpopular with some ethicists, it is enjoying something of a resurgence, but it is distinctly countercultural at the moment, gaining more attention as the poverty of ethical subjectivism becomes more manifest (Lisska 1996).

I do not claim to arrive at perfection in the grasp of moral truths. This can only be done asymptotically given the limitations of human intellect. But a realist approach is far less likely to miss the truth than some of the current more fashionable methods of philosophizing, which begin with the content of the mind rather than the world "out there."

These divergences notwithstanding, there are areas of fruitful interaction with existing models of ethics to which our approach can offer some insights.

For one thing, our system is consistent with principlism. To be sure, the notion of common morality is an insufficient foundation for a philosophy or ethic of medicine. The four principles, however, fit well with the kinds of obligations we would justify on the basis of the phenomena of medicine. Autonomy derives from a philosophical anthropology grounded in the inherent and essential dignity of every human being. Justice likewise would be the fulfillment of the moral claim of every human to fair and equal treatment. We would add the Aristotelian notion of *epikeia* to adjust justice to the particularities of a particular human being's life, thus addressing the difficulties of balancing principles when they are in conflict (Pellegrino 2002b).

We see hermeneutics and literature, now so popular not as independent theories of ethics but as important adjuvants to enable decision makers to comprehend their own and their fellow human experiences of the complexities and particular concrete details of the moral life. Narratives and hermeneutics are not normative per se but enhance our comprehension of the normative by their evocation of the concrete and detailed moral encounters that characterize every human life.

Feminism and caring we see also as important modulating influences on moral philosophy, raising sensitivities to long-neglected dimensions. But their normative claims, like all others, must pass philosophical muster. The same can be said of casuistry, dialogue, and dialectic. These are essential aspects of moral discourse and crucial to the resolution of conflicts since the first step must always be understanding the sources of conflict. But again they are not normative in themselves but helpful methodological aids to a realistically grounded moral philosophy.

We do not accept the powerful current conviction that, given the impossibility of moral consensus, we must abandon the search for the right and the good and instead be satisfied with what we can agree upon. This is simply another way to drive ethics as a discipline away from moral discourse and into "value" exchange and compromise. Values are personal attributions of worth or interest attached to things, ideas, or people. Being personal they are important and need to be taken account of in ethical discourse. But they are not by that fact norms, principles, duties, or obligations. It is a tribute to modern sensibilities that they occur in ethical discourse, but their limitations are also important to recognize.

Finally, I think that a philosophy of medicine and an ethic of the professions is crucial to the current move to reverse the trend toward deprofessionalization. Admirable as the effort may be, the recent "principles" and rules promulgated by the American Board of Internal Medicine, the American Society for Internal Medicine, and the European Federation of Internists are insufficient (Pellegrino 2001, 70–87; ABIM 2002, 243–46). Like the ancient Hippocratic oath, the current proposal is a set of moral and nonmoral assertions without an explicit moral foundation or justification. A deeper probing of what a profession is, what that entails morally, and what duties it requires is needed. This is true of the parallel efforts now extant in law, ministry, and teaching to "recapture" the idea of professional commitment. Without a reconstruction of the moral foundations of the idea of a profession, these efforts cannot be fully successful. They cannot succeed without clarity of their deeper moral underpinnings.

To be sure, reaffirmation of professionalism in the best sense is a necessary step in reprofessionalization. But the illness is now too deeply seated to be healed without a moral conception of what a profession entails and what makes it different from other occupations. We need much more careful consideration of what makes the professions sufficiently different to warrant designation of a special domain called "professional ethics."

The answer will not be found in constructing a "new" ethic for each profession. Such an exercise usually ends in manipulating long-standing moral precepts, converting duties and virtues into "values" and reformulating them in terms more palatable to modern tastes for "choice," private interpretations, and an atomized morality. When professional ethics becomes only what we can agree on or what we ourselves dictate, it becomes merely self-justifying. This is just as perilous as the older tendency to justify morality on the fact that the profession has defined it in a certain way. Professional codes must ground their authority and binding power in moral reality, not in professional privilege or preference.

We need to return to serious reflection on the nature of the good, the telos of professional activity, and the way both are related to the realities of human beings in predicaments of particular need. No enterprise could be more important in a world in which professional expertise plays so influential a role in the lives of all of us. Sooner or later, no matter what our own expertise may be, we all find ourselves in need of the help of some other professional. As soon as we step outside the narrow perimeter of our own expertise we are vulnerable to the ethical standards and character of those whom we consult.

Professional ethics, its groundings, the sources of its moral authority, and the way they are justified are of concern to all of us. It is not the whole of bioethics to be sure. But it is through professionals that bioethics becomes a benefit or a danger for every human being in a technological society. A philosophy of the profession that grounds the ethics of the professions is therefore more than an idle academic exercise.

The pathway of my scholarly interests has led me from medical ethics as a moral system based in an affirmation of certain moral precepts, to a search for the philosophical foundations of those precepts in a philosophy of medicine derived from the realities of medical practice, to a moral philosophy of healing. Such a moral philosophy has certain foundations common to all healing and helping professions. A better understanding of the moral foundations is essential to any definition of what constitutes a profession and distinguishes it from mere professionalism.

NOTES

I have understood the task assigned to me as a contributor to this volume to be a description of how my own thinking about the philosophy and ethics of medicine developed during the two decades of my association with the Kennedy Institute of Ethics. This has occasioned an inordinate concentration on my own writing. I trust this does no injustice to my colleagues.

1. For a more considered statement of my concerns about the future of bioethics, I refer you to a recent paper published in the *Journal of Medicine and Philosophy* (Pellegrino 2000, 655–75). For a look at the direction my work is taking from the philosophy of medicine as a basis of medical ethics, to a philosophy and moral philosophy of the health professions and the professions of law, ministry, and teaching, see my paper published in 2002 in the *Journal of Medicine and Philosophy* (Pellegrino 2002a, 556–79).

REFERENCES

ABIM Foundation, ACP-ASIM Foundation, and European Federation of Internal Medicine. 2002. Medical Professionalism in the New Millennium: A Physician Charter. *Annals of Internal Medicine* 136 (3): 243–46.

Jaspers, Karl. 1963. *Philosophy and the World, Selected Essays*. Washington, D.C.: Regnery.

Lisska, Anthony J. 1996. *Aquinas' Theory of Natural Law: An Analytic Reconstruction*. New York: Oxford University Press.

McElhinney, Thomas K., and Edmund D. Pellegrino. 2001. The Institute on Human Values in Medicine: Its Role and Influence in the Conception and Evolution of Bioethics. *Theoretical Medicine* 22: 291–317.

Pellegrino, E. D. 1966. Medicine, Philosophy, and Man's Infirmity in Conditio Humana. In *Edwin Straus on His Seventy-fifth Birthday*, edited by Walter von Baeyer and Richard M. Griffith. New York: Springer.

———. 1976. Philosophy of Medicine, Problematic and Potential. *Journal of Medicine and Philosophy* 1: 5–31.

———. 2000. Bioethics at Century's Turn: Can the Normative Be Retrieved? *Journal of Medicine and Philosophy* 25: 655–75.

———. 2001. Professional Codes. In *Methods in Medical Ethics*, edited by Jeremy Sugarman and Daniel Sulmasy. Washington, D.C.: Georgetown University Press.

———. 2002a. The Internal Morality of Clinical Medicine: A Paradigm for the Ethics of the Helping and Healing Professions. *Journal of Medicine and Philosophy* 26: 556–79.

————. 2002b. Rationing Health Care: Inherent Conflicts within the Concept of Justice. In *The Ethics of Managed Care: Professional Integrity and Patient Rights*, edited by William Bondeson and H. T. Engelhardt, Jr. Dordrecht: Kluwer.

Pellegrino, E. D., and D. C. Thomasma. 1981. *A Philosophical Basis of Medical Practice: Toward a Philosophy and Ethic of the Healing Professions.* Oxford: Oxford University Press.

————. 1987. *For the Patient's Good: The Restoration of Beneficence in Health Care.* Oxford: Oxford University Press.

————. 1993. *The Virtues in Medical Practice.* Oxford: Oxford University Press.

————. 1996. *The Christian Virtues in Medical Practice.* Washington, D.C.: Georgetown University Press.

————. 1997. *Helping and Healing: Religious Commitment in Health Care.* Washington, D.C.: Georgetown University Press.

Seifert, Josef. 1984. Essence and Infinity: A Dialogue with Existential Thomism. *The New Scholasticism* 58: 84–98.

Straus, Erwin. 1963. *The Primary World of Senses, A Vindication of Sensory Experience*, translated by Jacob Needleman. New York: The Free Press of Glencoe.

Von Hildebrand, Dietrich. 1973. *What Is Philosophy?* London and New York: W. Kohlhammer.

2

The Origins, Goals, and Core Commitments of *The Belmont Report* and *Principles of Biomedical Ethics*

TOM L. BEAUCHAMP

During the summer and the latter half of 1975, Jim Childress and I lectured on and began to write the chapters of what would later be titled *Principles of Biomedical Ethics*.[1] We worked steadily on this project throughout 1976. On December 22 of that year, I agreed to join the staff of the National Commission for the Protection of Human Subjects of Biomedical and Behavioral Research. My first and only major assignment was to write "The Belmont Paper," as it was then called—only later would it be titled *The Belmont Report*.[2]

There has been some confusion as to the historical origins of and connection between *Belmont* and *Principles*. Virtually all published commentary on this history has assumed that *Belmont* preceded and provided the abstract framework for *Principles*.[3] Such speculation about origins fails to appreciate that both works were written simultaneously, the one inevitably influencing the other. I will explain how this occurred. I will also defend the importance of general frameworks of moral principles of the sort found in these works against various criticisms that have appeared over the years.

THE ROOTS, DRAFTING, AND EVOLUTION OF *THE BELMONT REPORT*

The idea for the Belmont Paper originated in an examination of principles that emerged during a break-out session at a retreat held February 13–16, 1976, at the Smithsonian Institution's Belmont Conference Center.[4] This retreat predates my work on *The Belmont Report*, and I leave it to others to detail what transpired at Belmont.

A few months after this retreat, I received two phone calls, the first from Stephen Toulmin, then staff philosopher at the National Commission, and the second from Michael Yesley, staff director. They asked me to write a paper on the nature and scope of principles of justice for the commission, whose members, they thought, needed help in understanding theories and principles of justice and their application to moral problems of human subjects research. I wrote this paper and assumed that my work for the commission was concluded.[5]

However, shortly after I submitted the paper, Toulmin returned to full-time teaching at the University of Chicago, and Yesley inquired whether I would replace him on the commission staff. This appointment met resistance. Two commissioners who later became close friends of mine, Joe Brady and Donald Seldin, were less than enthusiastic about Yesley's nominee. Brady, who had built his reputation on research with monkeys, had heard me (together with LeRoy Walters) give a talk at Walter Reed on research involving animals, and he was unmoved by its content—or, rather, he was moved to a set of antagonistic comments. Seldin did not crave a youthful philosopher six years out of graduate school. He would have preferred John Rawls, or at least someone with an international reputation. Nonetheless, Yesley prevailed, likely with the help of chairperson Kenneth Ryan and my colleague and friend Patricia King, and I joined the commission staff (facilitated by a sabbatical leave from Georgetown).

I said that my first and only major assignment was to write the Belmont Paper. Here is how it came about: On my first morning in the office,[6] Yesley told me that he was assigning me full-time to writing this paper. I asked Yesley what the task was. He pointed out that the commission had been charged by Congress to investigate the ethics of research and to *explore basic ethical principles* (*The National Research Act* 1974).[7] Members of the staff were at work on various topics in research ethics, he said, but no one was working on basic principles. However, he continued, an opening round of discussions of the principles had been held at the Belmont retreat. The commission had delineated a rough schema of three basic ethical principles called "respect for persons," "beneficence," and "justice." I asked Yesley what these moral notions meant to the commissioners, to which he responded that he had no well-formed idea and that it was my job to figure out what the commissioners meant—or perhaps to figure out what they should have meant.

So, I found myself with the job of giving shape and substance to something called the Belmont Paper, though at that point I had never heard of Belmont or the paper. It struck me as a most odd title for a publication. Moreover, this document had never been mentioned during my interview for the job, or at any other time until Yesley gave me the assignment. My immediate sense was that I was the new kid on the block and had been given the dregs. When I decided to join the commission staff, I thought I was going to be working on the ethics of psychosurgery and research involving children—heated and perplexing controversies at the time. I was chagrined to learn that I was to write something on which no one else was working and that had its origins in a retreat I had not attended. Moreover, the mandate to do the work had its roots in a federal law that I had not until that morning seen or heard of.

Yesley proceeded to explain that no one had yet worked seriously on the sections of the report on *principles* because no one knew what to do with the federal mandate. This moment of honesty was not especially heartening, but I was not discouraged either, because Childress and I were at that time substantially into the writing of our book, then emphasizing the role of theories and principles in biomedical ethics.[8] Furthermore, Yesley gave me some hope by saying that a crude draft of the Belmont Paper already existed, though a twinkle in his eye warned me not to expect too much. So that morning (January 10, 1977) I read the "Belmont draft."[9] Scarce could a new recruit have been more dismayed. So little was said about the principles that to call it a "draft" of a document on principles is like calling a dictionary definition an encyclopedia article. Some sections were useful, especially a few pages drafted by Robert Levine on the subject of "The Boundaries between Biomedical and Behavioral Research and Accepted and Routine Practice" (later revised and published as the first section of *The Belmont Report* under the subtitle "Boundaries between Practice and Research"), but this draft document had almost nothing to say about the principles that supposedly were its heart. In the next few weeks I threw away virtually everything in this draft (or talked Yesley and Barbara Mishkin into putting its content into other commission documents) either because it contained too little on principles or because it had too much on peripheral issues, such as the commission's mandate, appropriate review mechanisms, compensation for injury, national and international regulations and codes, research design, and other items that did not belong in the Belmont Paper. Except for Levine's section on boundaries, virtually everything in this draft was eliminated.[10]

Once the Belmont "draft" was left with nothing in the section on principles—supposedly the heart of the document—Yesley fastened on the idea that I might find the needed content from that massive compendium on research titled *Experimentation with Human Beings* (Katz 1972).

Drawn from sociology, psychology, medicine, and law, this book was then, and perhaps is still today, the most thorough single collection of materials on research ethics and law. Yesley told me in a friendly but firm manner that I should know everything in this book. After several days of reading this rich resource, I found that it offered virtually nothing of relevance on *principles*. The various codes and statements by professional associations found in this book had some connection with my task and the commission's objectives, but only a very distant one.[11]

Fortunately, Childress and I had gathered a collection of high-quality material on principles and theories, largely in the writings of philosophers, most notably W. D. Ross and William Frankena. The big difference between our work and the commission's, as I saw it, was less the basic principles than the subject matter under consideration. Childress and I had been working largely on issues in clinical ethics and health policy. We had worked relatively little on research ethics, which was the sole focus of the commission. I saw in my early conversations with Yesley that these two projects—*Principles* and *Belmont*—had many points of intersecting interest and could be mutually beneficial. Once this sank in, I began to be more inspired by the assignment.

I spent many weeks drafting material on principles and then revising the drafts in response to feedback from both staff members and commissioners.[12] Seldin encouraged me with as much vigor as he could muster (which was—and remains today—considerable) to make my drafts as philosophical as possible. Seldin wanted some Mill here, some Kant there, and the signature of in-depth philosophical argument sprinkled throughout the document. I tried this style, but other commissioners wanted a minimalist statement relatively free of the style of academic philosophy. Seldin, Yesley, and I ultimately relented,[13] and bolder philosophical defenses of the principles were gradually stripped from the body of *Belmont*. This occurred in part because the commissioners wanted a brief statement and could not agree on how to justify the principles, though the commissioners had no difficulty in agreeing on the principles themselves.

I must give credit to Yesley for a key organizing conception in this report. He and I were in almost daily discussion about the Belmont Paper. We spent many hours discussing the best way to develop the principles, to express what the commissioners wanted to say, and even how to sneak in certain lines of thought that the commissioners might not notice. One late afternoon we were discussing the overall enterprise. We discussed each principle, whether the principles were really independent, and how the principles related to the topics in research ethics under consideration by the commission. Yesley said, as a way of summarizing our reflections, "What these principles come to is really quite simple for our purposes: Respect for persons applies to informed consent, beneficence applies to risk-benefit assessment, and justice applies to the selection of subjects." Yesley had articulated the following abstract schema:

Principle of	*applies to*	*Guidelines for*
Respect for persons		Informed consent
Beneficence		Risk-benefit assessment
Justice		Selection of subjects

This schema may seem trifling; certainly it was already nascent in preexisting drafts of the report and in the commission's deliberations. But no one at that time had articulated the schema in precisely this way, and Yesley's summary was immensely helpful in peering through countless hours of discussion to see the underlying structure and commitment at work in the principles that were destined to be the backbone of *Belmont*. Yesley had captured what would soon become the major portion of the table of contents of this report, as well as the rationale of its organization. I then attempted to draft the document so that the basic principles could be "applied" to develop guidelines in specific areas, and could also serve as the *justification* of the guidelines.

In light of this schema a general strategy emerged for handling problems of research ethics, namely, that each principle made moral demands in a specific domain of responsibility for research. For example, the principle of respect for persons demands valid consent. Under this schema, the *purpose* of consent provisions is not protection from risk, as many earlier federal policies seemed to imply, but the protection of autonomy and personal dignity, including the personal dignity of incompetent persons incapable of acting autonomously, for whose involvement a duly authorized third party must consent.

I wrote the sections on principles in *The Belmont Report* on this model of each principle applying to a specific compartment or zone. Yesley gave me free rein in this drafting, although the drafts were subject to revisions and improvements made by commissioners and staff members. They were revised, sometimes heavily. Public deliberations in commission meetings were a staple source of ideas, but a few commissioners spoke to me or to Yesley about desired changes, and a few commissioners proposed changes to Assistant Staff Director Barbara Mishkin, who passed them on to me. Most of these suggestions were accepted and a serious attempt was made to implement them. In this respect the writing of this document was a joint product of commissioner-staff interactions. However, most of the changes by commissioners concerned small matters, and commissioners were rarely involved in making written changes.[14]

This way of stating the history may suggest that the document grew in size over time, but the reverse was true. The document was contracted over time. I wrote much more for the commission about respect for persons, beneficence, and justice than eventually found its way into *The Belmont Report*. As this material was eliminated, I would scoop up the reject pile and fashion it for *Principles of Biomedical Ethics*, which at this point (roughly the summer of 1977) was more than 75 percent complete. One might say that various late-written chunks of this book were fashioned from the more philosophical, but abjured parts of what I wrote for the commission, the parts that never found the light of day. Undoubtedly my work at the commission accounts for the significant percentage of material on research ethics found in the first edition of *Principles*.

The final wordsmithing of *The Belmont Report* was done by three people in a small classroom at the National Institutes of Health (NIH).[15] Al Jonsen, Stephen Toulmin, and I were given this assignment by the commission. Some who have followed the later writings of Jonsen and Toulmin on casuistry may be surprised to learn that throughout the commission's deliberations, as well as in this final drafting, Jonsen and Toulmin contributed significantly to the clarification of the *principles* in the report. Neither proposed that a strategy of using principles should be other than central to the commission's statement of its ethical framework. I once reviewed all the commission transcripts pertaining to *Belmont*, primarily to study the commission's method of treating issues in research ethics. I found that Jonsen and Toulmin had occasionally mentioned casuistry, but they clearly understood the commission's casuistry as consistent with its use of moral principles.

I will have more to say later about the casuistry of Jonsen and Toulmin, as well as their understanding of the commission. But first I need to say more about the historical and structural relationship between *Principles of Biomedical Ethics* and *The Belmont Report*.

THE ORIGINS OF *PRINCIPLES OF BIOMEDICAL ETHICS*

In early 1976, coincidentally at almost exactly the date of the Belmont retreat, Childress and I submitted a prospectus for our book to the Oxford University Press.[16] We had already developed a general conception of what later came to be called by some commentators "mid-level principles." I knew nothing about the National Commission when we developed these ideas. Paradoxically, Childress was more familiar with the commission's work than I, because he had written a contract paper for the commissioners at an earlier date than I had.

Once I grasped the moral vision of the National Commission, I could see that Childress and I had major substantive disagreements with the commission. The principles articulated in *The Belmont Report* are "three" principles with names bearing notable similarities to some names of principles that Childress and I were using and continued to use, but the two schemas of principles are far from constituting a uniform name, number, or conception of principles of biomedical ethics. Indeed, the two frameworks are not coherent with one another.

I thought at the time, and still do, that the commission was confused in the way it delineated the principle of respect for persons. It seemed to blend two independent principles: a principle of respect for autonomy and a principle of protecting and avoiding the causation of harm to incompetent persons. Furthermore, Childress and I both thought that we should stick to our already developed thesis that the principle of beneficence must be distinguished from the principle of nonmaleficence, though the commission failed to make any such distinction. This matter was connected to another problem that later came to bother me, namely, that the commission's vision of beneficence was too utilitarian. Consequently, the commission had inadequate internal controls in its moral framework to protect subjects against abuse when there was the promise of major benefit for other sick or disabled persons.

The view that Childress and I defended at the time, and still today, is this: Four clusters of moral principles best serve the purpose of an abstract framework of moral principles:

1. Respect for autonomy (respecting the decision-making capacities of autonomous persons).
2. Nonmaleficence (avoiding the causation of harm).
3. Beneficence (providing benefits and balancing benefits against risks).
4. Justice (fairness in the distribution of benefits and risks).

Respect for autonomy. Respect for autonomy is now a frequently mentioned moral principle in biomedical ethics. It is rooted in the liberal moral and political tradition of the importance of individual freedom and choice. In moral philosophy personal autonomy refers to personal self-governance: personal rule of the self by adequate understanding while remaining free from controlling interferences by others and from personal limitations that prevent choice. "Autonomy" thus means freedom from external constraint and the presence of critical mental capacities such as understanding, intending, and voluntary decision-making capacity.

To respect an autonomous agent is to recognize with due appreciation that person's capacities and perspective, including his or her right to hold certain views, to make certain choices, and to take certain actions based on personal values and beliefs. The moral demand that we respect the autonomy of persons requires that autonomy of action should not be subjected to control by others. This principle provides the basis for the right to make decisions, which in turn takes the form of specific autonomy-related rights.

Controversial problems with the principle of respect for autonomy, as with all moral principles, arise when we must interpret its significance for particular contexts and determine precise limits on its application and how to handle situations when it conflicts with other moral principles. Many controversies involve questions about the conditions under which a person's right to autonomous expression demands actions by others, and also questions about the restrictions society may rightfully place on choices by patients or subjects when these choices conflict with other values. If restriction of the patient's autonomy is in order, the justification will always rest on some competing moral principle such as beneficence or justice.

Nonmaleficence. Since the days of Hippocrates, physicians have avowed that they would do their patients no harm. Among the most quoted principles in the history of codes of medical ethics is the maxim *primum non nocere*: "Above all, do no harm." Similar ideas have been many times repeated in classical medical writings and codes, and there can be little doubt that many basic rules in the common morality are requirements to avoid causing a harm. They include rules such as: Do not kill; Do not cause pain; Do not disable; Do not deprive of pleasure; Do not cheat; and Do not break promises. Similar prohibitions are found across the literature of biomedical ethics, each grounded in the principle that intentionally or negligently caused harm is a fundamental moral wrong.

There are many issues of nonmaleficence in medicine—some involving blatant abuses of persons and others involving subtle and unresolved questions. Blatant examples of failures to act nonmaleficently are found, for example, in the use of psychiatry to classify political dissidents as mentally ill, thereafter treating them with harmful drugs and incarcerating them with insane and violent persons. More subtle examples are found in the use of medications for the treatment of aggressive and destructive patients. These common treatment modalities are helpful to many patients, but they can be harmful to others. Physicians can also cause harm when they fail to take an adequate history, prescribe an improper dosage of medicine, fail to monitor and treat side effects, and the like.

Beneficence. A no less central value in medicine is that the welfare of patients is the goal of health care. Medicine's context and justification are found in clinical diagnoses and therapies aimed at the promotion of health by cure or prevention of disease. General obligations in the moral life, as well as specific duties in professional ethics requiring positive assistance, may be clustered under the heading of "beneficence." The principle of beneficence requires us to help others further their important and legitimate interests, often by preventing or removing possible harms.

The basic roles and concepts that give substance to the principle of beneficence in medicine are as follows: The positive benefits the physician is obligated to seek involve the alleviation of disease and injury. The harms to be prevented, removed, or minimized are the pain, suffering, and disability of injury and disease. The range of benefits a physician may help provide include helping patients find appropriate forms of financial assistance and helping them gain access to health care or research protocols. Sometimes the benefit is for the patient, at other times for society. Presumably such acts are required when the benefits are substantial and can be provided with minimal risk to the physician; one is not under an obligation of beneficence in all circumstances of risk.

An analysis of beneficence, broadly conceived, could lead to utilitarian demands of sacrifice and extreme generosity in the moral life, for example, giving a kidney for transplantation or donating bone marrow. The precise scope or range of acts required by the obligation of beneficence therefore needs to be limited, but drawing a precise line has proved to be difficult. Fortunately, we do not need a resolution in the present context. That we are morally obligated on some occasions to benefit others, at least in professional roles such as medicine and research, is not controversial.

Ordinary moral intuitions, as well as the intuitions of physicians, often suggest that certain duties not to cause harm to others are more compelling than duties to benefit them. However, this hierarchical ordering is not sanctioned by either morality or ethical theory. A harm inflicted may be negligible or trivial, whereas the harm to be prevented may be substantial: Saving a person's life by a therapeutic intervention often outweighs the harms (as well as the disrespect for autonomy) caused by involuntary institutionalization. One of the motivations for separating nonmaleficence from beneficence is that they conflict when one must either avoid harm or bring aid—and cannot do both. If the weights of the two principles vary, there can be no mechanical rule asserting that one obligation must always outweigh the other.

Justice. A person has been treated justly if treated according to what is fair, due, or owed. For example, if equal political rights are due all citizens, then justice is done when those rights are accorded. The term *distributive justice* refers to fair, equitable, and appropriate distribution in society determined by justified norms of distribution that structure part of the terms of social cooperation. Usually this term refers to the distribution of primary social goods, such as economic goods and fundamental political rights. But burdens are also within its scope. Paying for forms of national health insurance is a distributed burden; Medicare checks and grants to do research are distributed benefits.

There is no single principle of justice. Somewhat like principles under the heading of beneficence, there are several principles, each requiring specification in particular contexts. Philosophers have also developed diverse theories of justice that provide material principles and that defend the choice of principles. These theories attempt to elaborate how people are to be compared and what it means to give people their due. Egalitarian theories of justice emphasize equal access to primary goods; libertarian theories emphasize rights to social and economic liberty; and utilitarian theories emphasize a mixed use of such criteria so that public and private utility are maximized. These three theories of justice all capture some of our intuitive convictions about justice, each with a different use of principles.

The role of managed care in biomedical practice has raised many issues of distributive justice in recent years. For example, which forms of mental suffering create legitimate claims for coverage by health insurance, and what is the role of the notion of "medical necessity" in making such determinations? Should there be a scale of copayment that varies according to a patient's income? These are essentially questions of fairness, and the obligations of justice created by our answers to them often intersect with moral principles.

To conclude, these four principles were never intended to form a full moral system or theory, only to provide a framework through which we can identify and reflect on moral problems. The framework is abstract and spare, and moral thinking and judgment must take account of other considerations as well. Abstract principles do not contain sufficient content to address the nuances of moral circumstances. Often the most prudent course is to search for more information about cases and policies, rather than to try to decide prematurely on the basis of either principles or some general theoretical analysis.

The differences between the philosophy in *Principles of Biomedical Ethics* and the commission's views in *The Belmont Report* have occasionally been the subject of published commentary.[17] Some commentators correctly see that we developed substantially different moral visions, and that neither approach was erected on the foundations of the other. So, why did I not attempt to correct the commission's views, given that I had responsibility for drafting *Belmont*? By mid-1977 I had come to the view that the commission, especially in the person of its chair, Kenneth Ryan (and also Commissioner Karen Lebacqz and others), was sufficiently rigid in the commitment made to its interpretation of the principles that there was no way to substantially alter the commission's statement of principles, though I thought that all three principles were either defective or under-analyzed in one way or another.

It is, then, *structurally* inaccurate to say that Childress and I were adopting, amplifying, or developing the same principles as those of the commission; and it is *historically* inaccurate to state that either framework of principles was prior. There was reciprocity in the drafting, but the influence ran bilaterally. I was often simultaneously drafting material on the same principle or topic for both the commission and Childress; and Childress was at the same time writing material for me to inspect. I would routinely write parts of *The Belmont Report* during the day at commission headquarters on Westbard Avenue in Bethesda, then go to my office at Georgetown in the evening and draft parts of chapters for Childress to review. He would critique my work in the next few days and suggest changes. Our work on the book thus influenced how I drafted the Belmont document, and the converse. Despite their entirely separate beginnings, these projects grew up and matured together.[18]

THE EVOLUTION OF *PRINCIPLES* OF *BIOMEDICAL ETHICS*

Today *Principles of Biomedical Ethics* bears only a distant resemblance to its embodiment in the first edition, because over the years Childress and I have branched out from and developed our core views. In the parts of the book that deal with ethical theory, two primary developments and sources of influence are apparent. The first is our adoption, almost wholesale, of Henry Richardson's account of the specification of moral norms (Richardson 1990, 279–310; 2000, 285–307).[19] Though I will not discuss problems of specification here, Richardson's theory has had a profound impact on our conception of methodology.

Second, we developed the idea that the four principles are not philosophical constructs but rather are norms already embedded in public morality—a universal common morality. In this respect the norms are presupposed in the formulation of public and institutional policies. I believe that we were the first writers in bioethics to adopt this view of the common morality, though we were influenced at the time by the work of Alan Donagan (1977). Our view was and remains that persons who are serious about living a moral life know and do not question these core dimensions of morality. They know not to lie, not to steal property, to keep promises, to respect the rights of others, and not to kill or cause harm to innocent persons. No more basic moral norms exist than principles requiring that we respect persons, take account of their well-being, and treat them fairly. All persons serious about morality know not to violate these norms unless they have a morally good reason for doing so.

Over the years the moral epistemology on which I have settled is that we are morally *certain* about the principles in the common morality, but quite *uncertain* about (and in open disagreement about) particular specifications of them. I appreciate that *certainty* is rare in the moral life, and I mean to distinguish it sharply from the kind of psychological *certitude* that results from enculturation. Debate about the established norms of the common morality would be a waste of time in any culture.[20] If I am right, then the common morality is not merely one morality that differs from the plurality of moralities embraced by individuals and communities. In short, the common morality contains universally valid precepts that bind all persons in all places, albeit through *prima facie principles* (another dominant theme in *Principles of Biomedical Ethics*).

A principle, in our account, is a fundamental standard of conduct from which many other moral standards and judgments draw support, standing, and specification. For example, core professional duties can be delineated on the basis of basic moral principles. A problem often advanced against our account of principles is that a scheme of multiple, prima facie principles fails to handle conflict among the principles themselves. Allegedly, our account cannot resolve conflicts and controversies, and may even promote controversy by allowing irresolvable conflict. Some of our critics have claimed to surmount this problem with their own theories, but how they do so has never been made clear to me. I have yet to find a plausible theory of moral norms that does not in the end rest on a structure of prima facie principles.

A distinction is needed here between "morality" that is *universal* in the way I am suggesting, and "morality" that is *particular* to cultures, institutions, and even individuals. The universal principles of the common morality comprise only a skeletal body of moral standards. A broader account of morality includes ideals and attitudes that spring from particular cultures, religions, and institutions. Childress and I have never claimed otherwise, and I do not believe that it is possible to develop a theory that dodges this problem.

If we could be confident that some philosopher's moral theory was a better source for codes and policies than the universal principles of the common morality, we could work constructively on practical and policy questions by progressive specification of the norms in that theory. At present, we have no such theory, and even proponents of the same type of general theory typically disagree about its commitments, how to apply it, and how to address specific issues. The general norms and schemes of justification found in philosophical ethical theories are invariably more contestable than the norms in the common morality. We therefore cannot reasonably expect that a contested moral theory will be better for practical decision making and policy development than the morality that serves as our common heritage. This is an absolutely central thesis in *Principles* in its later, though not its earlier, editions.

THE ROLE OF CASUISTRY

The recent rise of casuistry has caused various misunderstandings of both *Principles* and *Belmont*. Some commentators have overread the commission's work as fundamentally a casuistry, and other commentators have underread *Principles* as competitive with—and possibly undermined by—casuistry. While the commission demonstrably used casuistical reasoning in its deliberations, its commitment to basic principles was never diminished as a result. Similarly, Childress and I have from our first edition used casuistical reasoning in the treatment of cases, but there is no inconsistency between this form of reasoning and a commitment to principles.

The casuistic method begins with cases whose moral features and conclusions have already been decided and then compares the salient features in the paradigm cases with the features of cases that require a decision. Analogical reasoning links one case to the next and serves as the primary model of moral reasoning (Jonsen and Toulmin 1988, 11–19, 251–54, 296–99; Jonsen 1991b, 299–302; Arras 1994, 983–1014).[21]

Defenders of casuistical reasoning see moral authority as analogous to the authority operative in case law: When the decision of a majority of judges becomes authoritative in a case, the judgments in their decision are positioned to become authoritative for other courts hearing cases with similar facts. As a history of similar cases and similar judgments mounts, a society becomes increasingly confident in its moral conclusions and acknowledges secure generalizations (that is, rules or principles) in its evolving tradition of ethical reflection.

Jonsen and Toulmin have argued that deliberations at the National Commission were rooted in a casuistry, rather than in universal principles or theory:

> The one thing [*individual* Commissioners] could not agree on was *why* they agreed. . . . Instead of securely established universal principles, . . . giving them intellectual grounding for particular judgments about specific kinds of cases, it was the other way around.
>
> The *locus of certitude* in the Commissioners' discussions . . . lay in a shared perception of what was specifically at stake in particular kinds of human situations. . . . That could never have been derived from the supposed theoretical certainty of the principles to which individual Commissioners appealed in their personal accounts. (Jonsen and Toulmin 1988, 16–19)

There is something right, but also something very misleading, about this interpretation. It is true that casuistical reasoning more than moral theory or universal abstraction forged agreement on hard cases during commission deliberations. The commissioners appealed to particular cases and families of cases, and consensus was reached through agreement on cases and generalization from cases.[22] It is also true that commissioners would never have been able to agree on a single ethical theory.[23]

Nonetheless, this methodological appraisal of commission deliberations is consistent with its firm commitment to moral principles. Commissioners, including Jonsen himself, were emphatic in their support of the general moral principles delineated in *The Belmont Report*, and they often made appeal to those principles to reinforce moral reasoning and conclusions reached about cases.[24] The transcripts of the commission's deliberations show a constant movement from principle to case, and from case to principle. Principles supported argument about how to handle a case; and precedent cases supported the importance of commitment to principles. Cases or examples favorable to one point of view were brought forward, and counterexamples were then advanced. Principles were invoked to justify the choice and use of both examples and counterexamples. On many occasions an argument was offered that a case judgment was irrelevant or immoral in light of the commitments of a principle.[25] The commission's deliberations and conclusions are best understood, then, as examples of reasoning in which principles become interpreted and specified by the force of examples and counterexamples. The same has been true of the arguments in *Principles of Biomedical Ethics* from the initial drafting of the work.

Despite what some commentators have assumed, it is doubtful that Jonsen ever intended to deny this understanding of principles and their roles, despite the widely held view that casuistry either dispenses with or competes with principles. Jonsen has explicitly said that "casuistic analysis does not deny the relevance of principle and theory" (Jonsen 1990, 65; Jonsen and Toulmin 1988, 10); and in a gloss on his own work, Jonsen has written:

> When maxims such as "Do no harm," or "Informed consent is obligatory," are invoked, they represent, as it were, cut-down versions of the major principles relevant to the topic, such as beneficence and autonomy, cut down to fit the nature of the topic and the kinds of circumstances that pertain to it. (Jonsen 1995, 244)

Jonsen goes on to point out that casuistry is "complementary to principles" and that "casuistry is not an alternative to principles: No sound casuistry can dispense with principles" (Jonsen 1995, 244–49).[26]

Casuists and those who support frameworks of principles like those in *Belmont* and *Principles* should be able to agree that when they reflect on cases and policies, they rarely have in hand *either* principles that were formulated without reference to experience with cases *or* paradigm cases lacking a prior commitment to general norms. It is hard to understand, then, why anyone would think of casuistry as a rival paradigm to principles. To move constructively from case to case or to attend to the relevant features of a particular situation, some stable guide to moral relevance must connect cases or situations. The rule is not part of the case or situation, but rather a way of interpreting and linking cases or situations. All analogical reasoning requires a connecting norm in order to show that one object or event is like or unlike another in relevant respects. The creation or discovery of these circumstance-linking norms cannot be achieved by analogy itself. Casuistry therefore presupposes at least rough-

and-ready principles, rules, or maxims as essential moral elements in the case.

Casuistry without principles presents a *method without content*—that is, a tool of thought that displays the fundamental importance of case-comparison and analogy in moral thinking but that lacks initial moral premises. It is certain that we reason morally by analogy almost daily, and we are often confident in our conclusions, but such analogies also often fail, and analogies themselves never warrant a claim of truth or certainty. This is why the common morality provides a vital substantive basis for moral thinking.

INTERNALIST CHALLENGES TO PRINCIPLES

Contemporary bioethics has often been concerned with whether the source that grounds and justifies conclusions in medical ethics is external or internal to medicine. A principlist approach suggests that the most basic moral standards are external to traditions of medical ethics and are universal standards. In contrast, various writers have developed either *internal* accounts or *mixed internal-external* accounts. Edmund Pellegrino and Tristram Engelhardt, in their very different ways, fit this description. Pellegrino defends an ethic derived from the ends of medicine, whereas Engelhardt (often joined in his work by Kevin Wildes) claims that distinct medical ethics have emerged from distinct cultural frameworks, each with internal norms that govern physicians. Neither writer, I believe, offers a sustainable alternative to the principlist approach that Childress and I defend.

Pellegrino's approach is an essentialist theory about the nature and end of medicine that is influenced by Aristotelianism. For him, medicine is "praxis and not theory" and "contains its end within itself":

> Once we have decided what medicine is and from that what kind of functions physicians perform, we can derive what they ought to do—that is, the content of medical ethics. I have suggested a reconstruction of medical morality of the interaction between three facets of the healing relationship—the fact of illness, act of profession, and . . . the right and good healing action for a particular patient. (Pellegrino 1983, 17, 21)

Pellegrino maintains that the end of medicine—healing—determines the obligations and virtues of the physician (Pellegrino 1998, 1999; Pellegrino and Thomasma 1981, chs. 8–9). However, Pellegrino denies that an internal morality of medicine is acceptable merely because it is traditional, customary, or sanctioned by medical associations (Pellegrino 1993, 1158–62). Physicians may not know the ends of medicine or may not promote them properly. Pellegrino insists that an internal medical morality must be faithful to the true end of medicine—that is, healing. He recognizes that physicians may have *goals* or *purposes* in medical practice that are not formally tied to the true end of medicine, but he views these goals too as external. State-ordered executions, abortions, forensic psychiatric evaluations, autopsies, circumcisions, and the rationing of life-support systems in ICUs would presumably be examples.

Pellegrino sometimes writes as if at least one *external* standard—beneficence—sits in judgment on all internal standards:

> We will contend that beneficence remains the central moral principle of the ethics of medicine. . . . Our aim is to redefine, and refine, the notion of beneficence in terms of the new practicalities and dimensions of the physician-patient relationship today. With the recent emergence in the medical ethics of the principle of autonomy, it seems necessary to strike a new balance between autonomy and beneficence, which to some ethicists seem to be in conflict. (Pellegrino and Thomasma 1988, 7–8)

Although this statement appears to incorporate an external, general standard of beneficence, Pellegrino views *medical* beneficence as an internal standard oriented exclusively to the end of healing (Pellegrino 1994, 362–64). This constraint on the scope of beneficence allows Pellegrino to limit what counts as a benefit for patients. The category of benefits cannot for him include, for example, providing reproductive controls or actively causing a merciful death.

This limitation on the scope of medical beneficence is critical to Pellegrino's program, but may also be its chief vulnerability. If beneficence is a general moral principle (and it is), and if physicians are positioned to supply many forms of benefit (and they are), then there is no manifest reason to tie physicians' hands or duties to the single benefit of *healing*. Patients and society may, with good reason, regard cosmetic surgery, sleep therapies, assistance in reproduction, genetic counseling, hospice care, physician-assisted suicide, abortion, sterilization, and other actual or potential areas of medical practice as important benefits that only physicians can safely and efficiently provide. These activities are not forms of healing, or at least it is unclear how they fit Pellegrino's prototype of healing. Moreover, healing and the benefits associated with it may be understood differently by different parties or cultures. What some view as beneficial healing, others may view as religiously proscribed interventions.

This problem is traceable to Pellegrino's thesis that healing is the sole end of medicine. He believes that he has provided a *real* definition of "medicine"—i.e., one that captures its true essence. I do not think, however, that it is possible to specify with precision on his model, or any model, where medicine ends and nonmedical activities begin. The concept of *medicine* is too ill-formed; and ordinary language, schools of medicine, and legal definitions all fail to provide exact boundaries. *Medicine* is a vague and inherently contestable concept.

Placement of a line to remedy this problem need not be arbitrary in particular contexts, because the stipulation of threshold points marking off the medical from the nonmedical can be accomplished for specific purposes such as insurance policies, health policies, and the curricula of medical schools. The problem is that each context will support a different threshold line from that drawn in another context. There will emerge no general reason to draw the line as Pellegrino does.

Pellegrino's vision of medicine, then, lacks a principled basis to exclude alternative accounts and disregards many benefits that physicians can and do provide that are of great importance to society and patients, including reproductive controls and technologies, withholding burdensome treatment, assistance in dying, the implementation of living wills, genetic testing, cosmetic surgery to improve appearance, preventive medicine, occupational medicine, epidemiology, health promotion, nutrition, relief of pain and suffering, and terminal care.

Engelhardt's approach, by contrast, incorporates elements of both internalism and externalism. It holds that an intractable secular moral pluralism pervades the modern world, causing moral commitments to be implemented in different ways in diverse cultures and groups (and even individual decisions). From this perspective, each community or group— not medical professionals or a universal end of medicine—provides standards external to medical institutions that determine its ends and how it will serve patients and the public. These local external standards are incorporated into the internal morality of medicine in every culture.

Engelhardt, together with Wildes, holds that profound disagreement exists about the nature of medicine and the requirements of medical ethics across communities such as Orthodox Judaism, Roman Catholicism, Hinduism, and secular humanism:

There is no way to discover either a canonical content-full secular morality or the correct morally content-full solutions to secular moral controversies. As a consequence, individuals meet as moral strangers when they are not bound by the communality of a shared moral vision that binds moral friends. Moral strangers do not see the world in the same way. . . . Moral strangers [cannot] resolve content-full moral controversies by sound rational argument. Moral friends, on the other hand, are individuals who do share such premises in common. (Engelhardt and Wildes 1994, 135–47, quote on p. 136; cf. Wildes 2000, 133, 137–40)

According to Engelhardt and Wildes, no universal morality of medicine spans particular communities or can be made to span them. Unique belief systems comprise "medical ethics." The outlook of Orthodox Judaism, for example, determines what is acceptable or unacceptable only for that portion of the Jewish nation and those steadfast physicians who accept its norms. Even concepts such as *medicine* and *healing* are defined by communities. What is considered a form of healing or care in one tradition may be proscribed in another. Examples are blood transfusions, resuscitation, organ transplantation, the use of fetal tissue, herbal medicine, etc. From this perspective, moral standards of what is obligatory and permissible in medicine *derive from the community, not from universal moral principles or universally shared ends of medicine*. Indeed, there are many medicines and correlative medical ethics, each with distinct objectives and internal principles.

Accordingly, any communally initiated system of care and any internal medical morality that conforms to it are morally as good as any other system of care and internal morality. All moral norms in these systems are worthy of respect, regardless of the principles that underlie them or the consequences of their adoption (Engelhardt and Wildes 1994, 137–38). These norms have moral authority if and only if they are accepted as authoritative by members of a community. The deep moral thesis at work in this account is skeptical: There are no substantive foundations in universal principles for a secular bioethics, and, lacking such foundations, there are no foundations of any sort of bioethics other than historical roots in communities (Engelhardt 1996, 105–24).

There are strengths but many weaknesses in this account. It is a defect that medical beneficence and social justice have no status in it except insofar as persons in a community have sanctioned such acts. This moral position can lead to shocking conclusions. For example, in this theory the community that taxes coercively to provide health care for the needy acts immorally (a sweeping conclusion that morally condemns effectively every existing national health care system); and the physician who beneficently stops the bleeding of an unconscious moral stranger on the street performs an impermissible act unless explicitly given permission to so act.

Engelhardt resists the tempting interpretation that his account is "simply a political theory" (Engelhardt 1996, 11), but it is difficult to locate moral substance beyond its political commitments. He himself denies that he presents a substantive moral point of view—i.e., a "content-full morality" (another underanalyzed notion in the theory). Indeed, he argues that his work presents a "purely procedural morality" that alone provides an adequate "account of the common morality that can bind moral strangers" (Engelhardt 1996, x, 9).

Whereas Pellegrino overemphasizes uniformity deriving from his single legitimate end of medicine—to the point of excluding dissimilarity of approach and legitimately different goals among medical practitioners— Engelhardt and Wildes make the opposite error. By overemphasizing diversity, they overlook basic similarities—that is, they neglect the core of near identical medical goals, interests, and shared morality among well-trained physicians from all cultural backgrounds. Physicians all over the world share goals and techniques of healing, palliation, rehabilitation, removing discomfort, diagnostic testing, and the like. There is shared moral viewpoint (however limited) and shared medical practice across these communities.

Paradoxically, Engelhardt also overstates the degree of shared agreement within "the communities of friends" that form the primary appeal and resource of his account. He envisions a cohesive, pervasively shared uniformity in each community, springing from a stable and reliable agreement over the nature of medicine and medical ethics. However, in many (perhaps all) communities of any size, there exists a pluralism of viewpoint. Rarely is a well-developed culture of medicine and medical ethics free of internal conflicts and controversies. These communities are not static and not lacking in subgroups with different moral points of view and hopes to revise prevailing conditions, practices, and codes. Changing circumstances of urbanization, education, industrialization, the evolution of civil rights, and the like make for fluid circumstances in these communities, and a consequent need to reassess their past norms and judgments.

Controversy tracks the growth and development of medicine even in highly unified communities. The thesis that prevailing rules of medical practice are justified and cement the bonds in these communities is a fragile proposition. I believe that there is no single culture in most of these communities and that this conclusion should be embraced by all who, like Engelhardt and Wildes, emphasize multiculturalism. The more medicine is beset with controversies such as those that surround abortion, sterilization, female circumcision, forensic psychiatry, cosmetic surgery, alternative medicines, innovative therapies, and commercialization of tissues and organs, the more there will be disagreement about legitimate ends and permissible means. This disagreement will occur *within* communities almost as commonly as *across* communities.

Another weakness is that Engelhardt's mixed internalist-externalist account effectively precludes cross-cultural—that is, cross-community—judgments. The validity of moral judgments depends in these theories on their endorsement by a community; no transcendent principle other than permission-giving is available to make cross-cultural appraisals and to foster conflict resolution (Engelhardt 1996, 57). Retrospective moral judgments suffer the same fate: We can judge a person as having performed a wrong action fifty years ago even though we now confidently conclude that this same action is right. For example, if fifty years ago it was morally wrong, according to some community, for a woman surgeon to perform surgery on a man, but today it is acceptable, then we can only judge actions in this community in accordance with the standards prevalent at the time they were performed. Fifty years ago it was wrong; today it is right.

It follows from Engelhardt's perspective that there are no universal human rights that protect physicians, patients, and subjects. Human rights are by definition valid claims that are justified by reference to morally relevant features of human beings—not by reference to communal standards. According to this perspective, a so-called *universal* right is merely a norm that is *contingently recognized* in all communities. Engelhardt does recognize—on the basis of an unclearly grounded universal obligation to abstain from force—the right to give permission for all medical interventions; but he concedes no other universal right (Engelhardt 1991, 126–38; 1996, 67–71, 83, 105, and ch. 8). There are no universal obligations or rights of justice or beneficence in his theory—e.g., no obligation that society construct a fair system of the distribution of cadaver organs, no right to medical treatment in an emergency circumstance, and no right to public health measures.

CONCLUSION

Moral "fundamentalism" in bioethics has recently been under attack as resting on the bankrupt idea that universal principles stand above the particular norms of particular cultures.[27] *The Belmont Report* and *Principles of Biomedical Ethics* have both been considered fundamentalist in the relevant sense of accepting fundamental principles that are universally applicable to clinical and research ethics.[28] Both works are fundamentalist about principles, though not in acceptance of a foundationalist ethical theory. Both works understand these principles as woven into the fabric of morality. If this is correct, then no responsible clinical practitioner or research investigator could, with moral integrity, treat patients or conduct research without conforming to these principles.[29]

Both works discussed in this essay represent, in the final analysis, defenses of universal principles, but ones that allow for diversity in the ways principles are specified in local cultures and institutions. If these two works have made an enduring contribution in bioethics, this principled, universalist stance may define that contribution.

NOTES

1. Several books were published in 1976 that had some influence on the writing of *Principles* as it came to completion. These included Brody 1976; Veatch 1976; Gorovitz et al. 1976; and Veatch and Branson 1976.

2. National Commission 1978b. See also *Appendices I and II to The Belmont Report* (National Commission 1978a). *The Belmont Report* was completed in late 1977 and published officially on September 30, 1978. It appeared officially in the *Federal Register* on April 18, 1979. To compare the dating, *Principles of Biomedical Ethics* was in near final form in late 1977, published in late 1978 with a 1979 copyright date.

    The National Commission for the Protection of Human Subjects of Biomedical and Behavioral Research was established July 12, 1974, under the National Research Act, Public Law 93-348, Title II. The first meeting was held December 3–4, 1974. The forty-eighth and final meeting was held September 8, 1978.

3. See, for example, Meslin et al. 1995, 399, 401, 403; Gert, Culver, and Clouser 1997, 72–74; and Moreno 1995, 76–78. Meslin et al. say that "Beauchamp and Childress's *Principles of Biomedical Ethics* . . . is the most rigorous presentation of the principles initially described in the *Belmont Report*" (403). Gert, Culver, and Clouser see *Principles* as having "emerged from the work of the National Commission" (73). Moreno presumes that Beauchamp and Childress "brought the three [Belmont] principles into bioethical analysis more generally."

    The thesis that the idea of an abstract framework of principles for bioethics originated with the National Commission has been sufficiently prevalent that authors and lecturers have occasionally cited the principles *as Childress and I have named and articulated them*, and then felt comfortable in attributing *these same principles* to the National Commission.

4. See the archives of Meeting 15, vol. 15A (February 13–16, 1976), prepared for the Belmont meeting. This meeting book contains a "staff summary" on the

subject of "ethical principles" as well as expert papers on ethics prepared by Kurt Baier, Alasdair MacIntyre, James Childress, Tristram Engelhardt, Alvan Feinstein, and LeRoy Walters. The papers by Engelhardt and Walters most closely lay out the kinds of considerations ultimately treated in the Belmont Paper, but neither quite landed on the National Commission's three principles. However, Walters came very close to a formulation of the areas to which the commission *applies* its principles.

5. The paper was eventually published as "Distributive Justice and Morally Relevant Differences," in *Appendix I to The Belmont Report*, pp. 6.1–20. This paper was distributed at meeting 22 of the National Commission, held in September 1976—seven months after the retreat at the Belmont Conference House.

6. The Saturday meeting of the commission on January 8, 1977, was my first day on the job. Yesley and I met the following Monday.

7. Congress charged the commission with (1) recommending regulations to the Department of Health, Education, and Welfare (DHEW) to protect the rights of research subjects and (2) developing ethical principles to govern the conduct of research. In this respect, *The Belmont Report* was at the core of the tasks the commission had been assigned by Congress. DHEW's conversion of its grants administration *policies* governing the conduct of research involving human subjects into formal *regulations* applicable to the entire department was relevant to the creation of the National Commission. In the U.S. Senate, Senator Edward Kennedy, with Jacob Javits's support, was calling for a permanent, *regulatory* commission independent of NIH to protect the welfare and rights of human subjects. Paul Rogers in the House of Representatives supported NIH in advocating that the commission be *advisory* only. Kennedy agreed to yield to Rogers if DHEW published satisfactory regulations. This compromise was accepted. Regulations were published on May 30, 1974; then, on July 12, 1974, P.L. 93-348 was modified to authorize the National Commission as an advisory body. Charles McCarthy helped me understand this history. For a useful framing of the more general regulatory history, see Brady and Jonsen (two commissioners) 1982, 3–18.

8. Childress and I had been working in areas of practical ethics for several years with an interest in the connection between theory, principles, and practical decision making and policy. His work had been centered in areas that we would bring together under the label of justice, and I had developed a special interest in the area we called respect for autonomy. These "principles" were already part of our working scheme before we encountered the National Commission's principles (as were nonmaleficence and beneficence).

9. This draft had a history beginning with a document prepared for Meeting 16 (March 12–14, 1976). This document, dated March 1, 1976, and titled "Identification of Basic Ethical Principles," summarized the relevant historical background and, most importantly, set forth the three "underlying ethical principles" that came to form the commission's framework. Each principle was discussed in a single paragraph. This document was slightly recast in a draft of June 3, 1976, prepared for Meeting 19 (June 11–13, 1976), but the discussion of principles was actually shortened to little more than one page devoted to all three principles.

Surprisingly, in the summary statement (p. 9), "respect for persons" was presented as the principle of "autonomy." No further draft was presented to the commission until ten months later, at Meeting 29 (April 8–9, 1977). I began work on the document in January 1977.

10. Cf. the radical differences between the draft available at Meeting 19 (June 11–13, 1976) and the draft at Meeting 29 (April 8–9, 1977). These drafts show unmistakably that the critical period during which the Belmont principles took shape was between January 1, 1977, and April 1, 1977. Many smaller improvements were made between April 1977 and the report's publication more than a year later. Of particular interest is the draft of December 2, 1977 (presented at Meeting 37), which at the time showed many similarities to the first edition of *Principles of Biomedical Ethics*. Childress and I had virtually completed our manuscript by this date, but the revising of *Belmont* would be taken through five more drafts presented to the commissioners, the last being presented at Meeting 43, the final meeting (September 8, 1978). By this time, Childress and I were returning galleys for *Principles* to Oxford University Press. (The marketing form for the book was scheduled for completion on September 26, 1978; galleys arrived October 25, 1978.)

11. The first and only footnote in *The Belmont Report* to *sources* is a throwaway reference to this background reading. Typical materials that I examined during this period include: *United States* v. *Karl Brandt*, (1948–49); reproduced in part in Katz 1972, 292–306; American Medical Association 1946, 1090; and World Medical Assembly 1964. Less helpful than I had hoped was Beecher 1966, 135–36. For behavioral research I started with Golann 1970, 398–405; and American Psychological Association 1973.

12. Jonsen, a commissioner, reports in his *The Birth of Bioethics* (1998, 120) that I was "working with [Stephen] Toulmin on subsequent drafts" of *The Belmont Report* in 1977. This account is incorrect. Though I always sat next to Stephen and conversed with him about many subjects during meetings of the commission throughout 1977, we never drafted or revised anything together on *Belmont* during this period. Stephen was at the time assigned to a different project on recombinant DNA. Several features of Jonsen's account of events in 1977 lack accuracy.

13. Yesley was my constant critic, more so than anyone else. Seldin was my constant counsel, forever exhorting me to make the document more philosophically credible, only to confront a majority of commissioners who wanted a simple and streamlined document. And throughout it all, Patricia King taught me more about the commission than anyone else. It was she who helped me understand why a really philosophical document was not the desired result.

14. One meeting occurred in September 1977 when a small group of staff and commissioners gathered in the belvedere or rooftop study in Jonsen's home in San Francisco. The group in attendance attempted to revise the Belmont Paper for presentation at the next meetings during which commissioners were scheduled to debate it. Jonsen reports in *The Birth of Bioethics* (p. 103) that "the date is uncertain" of this meeting at his home. In fact, the date is the afternoon of September 21 through September 23, 1977. Jonsen also misremembers the group

of people present at the meeting. He correctly reports that the purpose of the meeting was to revisit "the February 1977 deliberations" of the commissioners, but he incorrectly reports in the same sentence that the meeting was called "to revise the June 1976 draft." Except for a section on boundaries written by Robert Levine, the June 1976 draft had long ago been so heavily recast that *Belmont* was by September 1977 a completely different document. Jonsen appears unaware that eight months of continual redrafting of *Belmont* had occurred (from February to September 1977) prior to the meeting at his home. On the one hand, this oversight is not surprising since the commission did not discuss the draft reports at its meetings during those eight months. On the other hand, new "staff drafts" of the Belmont Paper were distributed at two meetings during this period, namely, Meeting 29 (April 8–9, 1977) and Meeting 30 (May 13–14, 1977). All drafts are now housed in the archives of the Kennedy Institute Library.

15. Our wordsmithing meetings occurred on May 31–June 1, 1978, just prior to the commission's forty-second and penultimate meeting, on June 9–10, 1978. Thus, the wording at Meeting 42 would have been the final wording unless a commissioner raised an objection at that meeting or the next.

16. Initial plans for this book arose through a series of discussions in 1974–75 with Seymour Perlin, a psychiatrist then at the Kennedy Institute of Ethics and also at the George Washington University. Perlin helped draft the cover letter and prospectus for the book and promoted it with the Oxford University Press. After review of the completed work, the contract for the book was issued by the Oxford University Press on August 19, 1976, over four months before I went to work for the National Commission.

17. Particularly insightful on this topic is Marshall (1986, 5–6). See also Fletcher 1992, 95–121, esp. sect. IV, "Resources in Research Ethics: Adequacy of the Belmont Report."

18. For more on the nature and history of commitment to principles in bioethics, see Gert, Culver, and Clouser 1997, 72ff; Beauchamp and DeGrazia 2002; Childress 1994, 181–201; Beauchamp 1994a, 3–12; Beauchamp 1994b, 1–17; Beauchamp 1996; and Winkler 1996.

19. Specification requires reducing the indeterminateness of the general norms to give them increased action-guiding capacity, while retaining the moral commitments in the original norm. Filling out the commitments of the norms with which one starts is accomplished by narrowing the scope of the norms, not merely by explaining what the general norms mean. The scope is narrowed, as Richardson puts it, by "spelling out where, when, why, how, by what means, to whom, or by whom the action is to be done or avoided" (Richardson 2000, 289). See, further, DeGrazia 1992, 511–39; and Beauchamp and DeGrazia 2001, esp. 33–36.

   Some useful reflection on the limits of general principles and the need for their specification in frameworks like those of *Principles* and *Belmont* is found in Cassell 2000, 12–21; Macklin 1996, 183–98; Fulford and Hope 1994, 681–95; and Levine 1996, 105–26, esp. 106–9.

20. Although there is only a single common morality, there is more than one *theory* of the common morality. The common morality is universally shared; it is not a

theory of what is universally shared. A common-morality theory also does not hold that all *customary* moralities qualify as part of the *common* morality; and use of the common morality in moral reasoning need not lead to conclusions that are socially received. An important function of the general norms in the common morality is to provide a basis for the evaluation and criticism of groups or communities whose customary moral viewpoints are deficient.

21. See also Toulmin 1981, 31–39.

22. See, further, Toulmin 1987, 599–613; and Jonsen 1991a, 113–30.

23. Nor did they even attempt to buttress the *Belmont* principles with a specific theory. Jonsen and Toulmin's treatment of the National Commission is, in this regard, insightful and unobjectionable; and a similar line of argument can be taken to explicate the methods of reasoning at work in other bioethics commissions. See, for example, Capron 1983, 8–9.

24. See Jonsen's own summation to this effect in his "Casuistry" (2001, 112–13); and his introduction to *The Belmont Report* in Jonsen, Veatch, and Walters 1998, 22.

25. See National Commission, "Transcript of the Meeting Proceedings" for the following meetings: February 11–13, 1977, pp. 11–155; July 8–9, 1977, pp. 104–17; April 14–15, 1978, pp. 155–62; and June 9–10, 1978, pp. 113–19. These transcripts are archived in the Kennedy Institute Library.

26. See also Jonsen 1996, 59–82.

27. See, for example, the critique in Baker 1998a, 201–31; 1998b 233–74.

28. *The Belmont Report* makes reference to "our cultural tradition" as the basis of the principles (p. 4). Robert Levine pointed out at the time the *Report* was published that an early draft of the *Report* contained language indicating that the commission was relying on "three fundamental principles . . . consonant with the major traditions of Western ethical, political, and theological thought represented in the pluralistic society of the United States" (Levine 1981, 9, quoting his own 1978 paper and an early draft of *The Belmont Report*). Cf. Moreno's interpretation (1995, 76) of the background and evolution of the principles.

29. For a commission that explicitly supports a fundamentalist set of principles, see Advisory Committee on Human Radiation Experiments (ACHRE) 1996, esp. ch. 4.

References

Advisory Committee on Human Radiation Experiments (ACHRE). 1996. *Final Report of the Advisory Committee on Human Radiation Experiments.* New York: Oxford University Press.

American Medical Association, House of Delegates, Judicial Council. 1946. Supplementary Report of the Judicial Council. *Journal of the American Medical Association* 132: 1090.

American Psychological Association, Inc. 1973. *Ethical Principles in the Conduct of Research with Human Participants.* Washington, D.C.: APA.

Arras, John. 1994. Principles and Particularity: The Role of Cases in Bioethics. *Indiana Law Journal* 69: 983–1014.

Baker, Robert. 1998a. A Theory of International Bioethics: Multiculturalism, Postmodernism, and the Bankruptcy of Fundamentalism. *Kennedy Institute of Ethics Journal* 8: 201–31.

———. 1998b. A Theory of International Bioethics: The Negotiable and the Non-Negotiable. *Kennedy Institute of Ethics Journal* 8: 233–74.

Beauchamp, Tom. 1994a. The Four Principles Approach to Medical Ethics. In *Principles of Health Care Ethics*, edited by R. Gillon. London: John Wiley & Sons.

———. 1994b. Principles and Other Emerging Paradigms for Bioethics. *Indiana Law Journal* 69 (3): 1–17.

———. 1996. The Role of Principles in Practical Ethics. In *Philosophical Perspectives on Bioethics*, edited by L. W. Sumner and J. Boyle. Toronto: University of Toronto Press.

Beauchamp, Tom, and James Childress. 1978. *Principles of Biomedical Ethics.* 1st ed. New York: Oxford University Press.

———. 2001. *Principles of Biomedical Ethics.* 5th ed. New York: Oxford University Press.

Beauchamp, Tom, and David DeGrazia. 2001. Philosophical Foundations and Philosophical Methods. In *Methods in Medical Ethics*, edited by J. Sugarman and D. Sulmasy. Washington, D.C.: Georgetown University Press.

———. 2002. Principlism. In *Bioethics: A Philosophical Overview* (volume I of *Handbook of the Philosophy of Medicine*), edited by George Khusfh. Dordrecht: Kluwer.

Beecher, Henry. 1966. Some Guiding Principles for Clinical Investigation. *Journal of the American Medical Association* 195: 1135–36.

Brady, Joseph V., and Albert R. Jonsen. 1982. The Evolution of Regulatory Influences on Research with Human Subjects. In *Human Subjects Research*, edited by Robert Greenwald et al. New York: Plenum Press.

Brody, Howard. 1976. *Ethical Decisions in Medicine.* Boston: Little, Brown and Co.

Capron, Alexander. 1983. Looking Back at the President's Commission. *Hastings Center Report* 13 (5): 8–9.

Cassell, Eric J. 2000. The Principles of The Belmont Report Revisited: How Have Respect for Persons, Beneficence, and Justice Been Applied to Clinical Medicine? *Hastings Center Report* 30 (July/August 2000): 12–21.

Childress, James. 1994. Ethical Theories, Principles, and Casuistry in Bioethics: An Interpretation and Defense of Principlism. In *Religious Methods and Resources in Bioethics*, edited by Paul F. Caminisch. Boston: Kluwer.

DeGrazia, David. 1992. Moving Forward in Bioethical Theory: Theories, Cases, and Specified Principlism. *Journal of Medicine and Philosophy* 17: 511–39.

Donagan, Alan. 1977. *The Theory of Morality.* Chicago: University of Chicago Press.

Engelhardt, Tristram. 1991. *Bioethics and Secular Humanism*. Philadelphia: Trinity Press International.

———. 1996. *Foundations of Bioethics*. 2d ed. New York: Oxford University Press.

Engelhardt, Tristram, and Kevin Wildes. 1994. The Four Principles of Health Care Ethics and Post-Modernity. In *Principles of Health Care Ethics*, edited by R. Gillon. London: John Wiley & Sons.

Fletcher, John C. 1992. Abortion Politics, Science, and Research Ethics: Take Down the Wall of Separation. *Journal of Contemporary Health Law and Policy* 8: 95–121.

Fulford, K. W. M., and Tony Hope. 1994. Psychiatric Ethics: A Bioethical Ugly Duckling. In *Principles of Health Care Ethics*, edited by R. Gillon. London: John Wiley & Sons.

Gert, Bernard, Charles M. Culver, and K. Danner Clouser. 1997. *Bioethics: A Return to Fundamentals*. New York: Oxford University Press.

Golann, Stuart E. 1970. Ethical Standards for Psychology: Development and Revisions, 1938–1968. *Annals of the New York Academy of Sciences* 169: 398–405.

Gorovitz, Samuel, et al., eds. 1976. *Moral Problems in Medicine*. Englewood Cliffs, N.J.: Prentice Hall.

Jonsen, Albert. 1990. Case Analysis in Clinical Ethics. *The Journal of Clinical Ethics* 1: 65.

———. 1991a. American Moralism and the Origin of Bioethics in the United States. *Journal of Medicine and Philosophy* 16: 113–30.

———. 1991b. Casuistry as Methodology in Clinical Ethics. *Theoretical Medicine* 12: 299–302.

———. 1995. Casuistry: An Alternative or Complement to Principles? *Kennedy Institute of Ethics Journal* 5: 237–51.

———. 1996. The Weight and Weighing of Ethical Principles. In *The Ethics of Research Involving Human Subjects: Facing the Twenty-first Century*, edited by Harold Y. Vanderpool. Frederick, Md.: University Publishing Group.

———. 1998. *The Birth of Bioethics*. New York: Oxford University Press.

———. 2001. Casuistry. In *Methods in Medical Ethics*, edited by Jeremy Sugarman and Daniel P. Sulmasy. Washington, D.C.: Georgetown University Press.

Jonsen, Albert, and Stephen Toulmin. 1988. *The Abuse of Casuistry*. Berkeley: University of California Press.

Jonsen, Albert, Robert M. Veatch, and LeRoy Walters, eds. 1998. *Source Book in Bioethics*. Washington, D.C.: Georgetown University Press.

Katz, Jay, with the assistance of Alexander Capron and Eleanor Glass, eds. 1972. *Experimentation with Human Beings*. New York: Russell Sage Foundation.

Levine, Robert J. 1981. *Ethics and Regulation of Clinical Research*. 1st ed. Baltimore: Urban & Schwarzenberg.

Levine, Carol. 1996. Changing Views of Justice after Belmont: AIDS and the Inclusion of "Vulnerable Subjects." In *The Ethics of Research Involving Human Subjects:*

Facing the Twenty-first Century, edited by Harold Y. Vanderpool. Frederick, Md.: University Publishing Group.

Macklin, Ruth. 1996. Trials and Tribulations: The Ethics of Responsible Research. In *Pediatric Ethics: From Principles to Practice*, edited by Robert C. Cassidy and Alan R. Fleischman. Amsterdam, Netherlands: Harwood Academic Publishers.

Marshall, Ernest. 1986. Does the Moral Philosophy of the Belmont Report Rest on a Mistake? *IRB: A Review of Human Subjects Research* 8: 5–6.

Meslin, Eric, et al. 1995. Principlism and the Ethical Appraisal of Clinical Trials. *Bioethics* 9: 399–418.

Moreno, Jonathan D. 1995. *Deciding Together: Bioethics and Consensus*. New York: Oxford University Press.

National Commission for the Protection of Human Subjects of Biomedical and Behavioral Research. Archived Materials 1974–78. "Transcript of the Meeting Proceedings" (for discussion of the Belmont Paper at the following meetings: February 11–13, 1977; July 8–9, 1977; April 14–15, 1978; and June 9–10, 1978). All archived material is at the Kennedy Institute Library, Car Barn storage facility, Georgetown University.

———. 1978a. *Appendices I and II to The Belmont Report: Ethical Guidelines for the Protection of Human Subjects of Research*. 2 vols. Washington, D.C.: DHEW Publication OS 78-0013 and OS 78-0014.

———. 1978b. *The Belmont Report: Ethical Guidelines for the Protection of Human Subjects of Research*. Washington, D.C.: DHEW Publication OS 78-0012.

The National Research Act, July 12, 1974. Public Law 93-348, Title II.

Pellegrino, Edmund. 1983. The Healing Relationship: The Architectonics of Clinical Medicine. In *The Clinical Encounter: The Moral Fabric of the Patient-Physician Relationship*, edited by E. Shelp. Dordrecht: D. Reidel.

———. 1988. *For the Patient's Good: The Restoration of Beneficence in Health Care*. New York: Oxford University Press.

———. 1993. The Metamorphosis of Medical Ethics: A Thirty-Year Retrospective. *Journal of the American Medical Association* 269: 1158–62.

———. 1994. The Four Principles and the Doctor-Patient Relationship: The Need for a Better Linkage. In *Principles of Health Care Ethics*, edited by R. Gillon. London: John Wiley & Sons.

———. 1998. The False Promise of Beneficent Killing. In *Regulating How We Die*, edited by L. L. Emanuel. Cambridge, Mass.: Harvard University Press.

———. 1999. The Goals and Ends of Medicine: How Are They to Be Defined? In *The Goals of Medicine*, edited by M. J. Hanson and D. Callahan. Washington, D.C.: Georgetown University Press.

Pellegrino, Edmund, and Thomasma, David. 1981. *The Philosophical Basis of Medical Practice*. New York: Oxford University Press.

Richardson, Henry S. 1990. Specifying Norms as a Way to Resolve Concrete Ethical Problems. *Philosophy and Public Affairs* 19: 279–310.

————. 2000. Specifying, Balancing, and Interpreting Bioethical Principles. *Journal of Medicine and Philosophy* 25: 285–307.

Toulmin, Stephen. 1981. The Tyranny of Principles. *Hastings Center Report* 11 (December 1981): 31–39.

————. 1987. The National Commission on Human Experimentation: Procedures and Outcomes. In *Scientific Controversies: Case Studies in the Resolution and Closure of Disputes in Science and Technology*, edited by H. T. Engelhardt Jr., and A. Caplan. New York: Cambridge University Press.

United States v. *Karl Brandt, Trials of War Criminals before the Nuremberg Military Tribunals under Control Council Law No. 10.* 1948–49. Military Tribunal I, Washington, D.C.: U.S. Government Printing Office. Vols. 1 and 2.

Veatch, Robert. 1976. *Death, Dying, and the Biological Revolution.* 1st ed. New Haven, Conn.: Yale University Press.

Veatch, Robert M., and Roy Branson, eds. 1976. *Ethics and Health Policy.* Cambridge, Mass.: Ballinger Publishing Co.

Wildes, Kevin. 2000. *Moral Acquaintances: Methodology in Bioethics.* Notre Dame, Ind.: University of Notre Dame.

Winkler, Earl. 1996. Moral Philosophy and Bioethics: Contextualism versus the Paradigm Theory. In *Philosophical Perspectives on Bioethics*, edited by L. W. Sumner and J. Boyle. Toronto: University of Toronto Press.

World Health Organization, 18th World Medical Assembly, Helsinki, Finland. 1964. Declaration of Helsinki: Recommendations Guiding Medical Doctors in Biomedical Research Involving Human Subjects. *New England Journal of Medicine* 271: 473–74.

3

Principles of Biomedical Ethics: Reflections on a Work in Progress

JAMES F. CHILDRESS

The subtitle of this chapter may be unsettling—"a Work in Progress" may suggest that yet another edition of *Principles of Biomedical Ethics* (hereafter *PBE*) is on the way. Perhaps there will be another edition, a sixth edition, but for now I will focus on some themes that, in my judgment, have been important as this work has evolved from our initial discussions to the present and on some issues that require further attention, in part to address critics' legitimate objections. It is probably unnecessary to note that these are *my* personal reflections and that Tom Beauchamp may have a very different interpretation.

I will use the term "principlism" as a shorthand expression for *PBE*'s framework. Even though the term "principlism" originated as a scornful label for our approach, it is useful because it is more succinct than, say, a "principles-based approach" or "the four-principles approach." Often a pejorative label becomes accepted and even used by those it derides. So I will use the label "principlism" in a neutral sense and with the understanding that it actually covers a variety of positions, not simply the one that *PBE* presents.

BACKGROUND TO *PRINCIPLES OF BIOMEDICAL ETHICS*

Tom Beauchamp and I knew each other at Yale Divinity School, where we both studied in the early 1960s, before he commenced his doctoral studies in philosophy at the Johns Hopkins University. As far as I can recall, we didn't meet again until I interviewed for the Joseph P. Kennedy, Sr., Professorship in Christian Ethics at the Kennedy Institute of Ethics in 1974. Then, after I accepted that appointment in 1975, we began discussing ethical theories, particularly because of his utilitarian and my deontological bent, and we started teaching together in the Intensive Bioethics Course (then called the Total Immersion Course) where we focused on debates about ethical theory. Obviously, our discussions benefited from many other conversation partners at the Kennedy Institute of Ethics, and I express my deep gratitude to them. One—psychiatrist Seymour Perlin—joined in our efforts to develop what became *Principles of Biomedical Ethics.* Other commitments prevented him from continuing to the end, but he arranged a meeting with Jeffrey House, an editor at Oxford University Press, which had previously published his *Handbook for the Study of Suicide* (Perlin 1975).

In looking over some files for this presentation, I discovered that we actually started our work on *Principles of Biomedical Ethics* earlier than I had recalled. In my files is a letter from Tom to Seymour Perlin and me dated December 7, 1975, in response to an outline of "possible topics" I had prepared, on the basis of our earlier discussions, and circulated to both of them. My earlier note to them had indicated that this draft of "Possible topics for volume with Perlin and Beauchamp" was "intended as a starting point, based on previous conversations, for our serious discussions." It had three basic sections: "Ethical Theory"; "Issues in Biomedical Ethics" (largely various principles and rules); and "Cases."

Then, after months of discussion, we submitted our formal proposal to Oxford University Press sometime in 1976: "We propose to write a general, distinctive, needed volume on biomedical ethics. . . . We would describe our project as a general book in biomedical ethics, both because it is intended to be comprehensive and because it is designed to meet a variety of needs. . . . It is introductory in the sense that it does not presuppose previous work in the field. Although it is more or less comprehensive in terms of identification of relevant moral notions and their applications to most types of cases (some, of course, in more detail than others), it is more than a survey of the field since it is systematically developed. Major alternative views will be identified, interpreted, and criticized at important points, but the volume is not intended to be a survey of all positions and issues." Later in the proposal we noted that our effort "stems from our frustration as teachers in undergraduate, graduate, and professional programs which need a basic textbook in biomedical ethics." We wanted to "cover the field in a systematic way" because virtually no books then available attempted to do so.

We further claimed in our proposal: "One distinctive and valuable feature of the volume is its integrated presentation of ethical theory. Rather than presenting biomedical ethics as a series of topical problems—

e.g., abortion, euthanasia, suicide, or genetic engineering—we combine [principles and cases]. The principles are used throughout the book to help resolve moral problems that arise in the cases and the cases in turn are used as tests of the adequacy of the principles." I will return to this point later.

By the time we submitted the proposal, the table of contents had further evolved. While the first section remained "Ethical Theory," and the third "Cases," the middle section was now titled "Principles of Biomedical Ethics," and that would eventually become the title for the book.

As might have been expected, we did not deliver on everything we promised in the proposal. Our colleague Seymour Perlin, as I noted earlier, was unable to continue the collaboration. And we promised much more attention to religious and quasi-religious perspectives than we actually delivered. We also continued to revise the structure, before finally settling on four principles with several derivative rules and with considerable attention to virtues and ideals (in the final chapter until the fifth edition) and numerous cases (twenty-nine) in the appendix.

PBE is genuinely a coauthored book. In the first edition we wrote: "This is a jointly authored book in every sense of the term. Although each author initially had primary responsibility for certain chapters [or sections of chapters], both authors rewrote substantial parts of every chapter and take responsibility for the whole, which at every point bears their dual imprint, whether by conviction or by compromise" (Beauchamp and Childress 1979, xiv). Our choice of initial primary responsibility for a chapter or section really reflects what we are most interested in at the time or have recently been exploring. Then it is up to the other to revise it and so forth. If one of us thinks that a section is seriously flawed, it is up to that person to produce a revision. And we keep exchanging revisions until we reach a version that is acceptable to both of us. We have not always achieved an overlapping consensus, and sometimes we let differences stand, for instance, by noting one author's preference. The collaboration works well because vigorous disagreements do not damage the collegial or personal relationships.

In my view, each edition of *PBE* participates in an ongoing conversation, not only between the coauthors but also with others in the field. We have tried to learn not only from our critics' specific objections and suggestions but also from quite different theories, perspectives, and frameworks. Indeed, after a period when, according to Dan Callahan and others, principlism was the dominant framework, various approaches have been vying for dominance for the last ten to fifteen years. Beginning in the fourth edition (which appeared in 1994) and continuing in the fifth edition (2001), we have tried to offer a critical analysis and evaluation of, as well as responses to, these various approaches, indicating as clearly as possible what we believe they contribute. So in the fourth edition, for each theory or framework, we prepared a section on "critical evaluation" and another on "constructive evaluation." This led to a tremendous expansion of the discussion of various approaches in the fourth edition and then to their relocation in the final chapters in the fifth edition, so that readers did not suppose they had to work through all of these theoretical and methodological arguments in order to use our own framework.

In short, we have been willing, even eager, to learn from various critical and alternative approaches, and to incorporate their insights, whenever possible, into our framework. Indeed, one friendly critic, my colleague John Arras, has suggested that our book is really like the Borg in *Star Trek*. Followers of *Star Trek*, which I am not, will recall the Borg, the half-machine, half-human creatures with a highly developed group consciousness (the "Borg Collective"). Each individual Borg is "linked by a sophisticated subspace network that constantly provides each member with supervision and guidance. Anyone captured by the Borg is automatically assimilated into the Collective" (Barad with Robertson 2001, 57). I would respond that, rather than capturing or assimilating various approaches, we try to learn from them, modifying and revising our framework as appropriate. One reason it is possible for me to summon the intellectual energy to work on yet another edition is the exciting challenge of taking account of important criticisms and then either trying to rebut them or trying to modify or revise our framework accordingly. This is the ongoing conversation that is so stimulating.

In this essay, I want to focus on the framework of principles/rules, with particular attention to the methodological and normative significance of community and the relation between principles/rules and cases, especially in specifying and balancing principles and rules.

COMMUNITY—ITS METHODOLOGICAL AND NORMATIVE SIGNIFICANCE

From Convergence to Common Morality

I will use the term "community" somewhat loosely to address two major issues in *PBE*, one methodological and the other substantive. First, methodologically, the early editions of *PBE* developed the four principles plus related rules out of a convergence or "overlapping consensus" between rule utilitarianism (Tom's favored theory) and rule deontology (my favored approach). We viewed these principles as shared requirements of adequate rule utilitarian and rule deontological theories. For instance, we drew on deontologist W. D. Ross, who in *The Right and the Good* recognized prima facie duties of fidelity; reparation; gratitude; justice; beneficence; nonmaleficence; and self-improvement (Ross 1930; see also Ross 1939). We emphasized the prima facie duties particularly relevant for actions in science, medicine, and health care, and added respect for autonomy, again because of its relevance in the context—principles of biomedical ethics. But we also drew on rule utilitarian Richard Brandt, who wrote:

> [The best set of rules] would contain rules giving directions for recurrent situations that involve conflicts of human interests. Presumably, then, it would contain rules rather similar to W. D. Ross's list of prima facie obligations; rules about the keeping of promises and contacts, rules about debts of gratitude such as we may owe to our parents, and, of course rules about not injuring other persons and about promoting the welfare of others where this does not work a comparable hardship on us. (Brandt 1968, 166)

Our argument for the four principles proceeded by elaborating the implications of adequate rule utilitarian and rule deontological approaches and their convergence, in line with Brandt (1979), Frankena (1973), and others.

But then in the fourth and fifth editions, we based our argument on "common morality," not on the convergence of these two types of ethical theory (even though we still recognized and affirmed this convergence). We emphasize that the common morality "comprises all and only those norms that all morally serious persons accept as authoritative" (Beauchamp and Childress 2001, 3). This is a metaethical thesis, not an empirical one. In addition, there are various communal moralities, that is, the communal norms, ideals, and virtues accepted by various particular communities. However, the common morality "establishes obligatory moral standards for everyone" (Beauchamp and Childress 2001, 4).

Community and Individuals:
The Normative Significance of Community(ies)

According to Ezekiel Emanuel, the shift to common morality in the fourth edition of *PBE* allows interpreters and critics to ask "whether other values, such as communal solidarity, ought to be incorporated as one of the values embedded in common morality" (Emanuel 1995). Similarly, at the first meeting of the National Bioethics Advisory Commission (NBAC) in October 1996, and with specific reference to research involving human subjects, Emanuel contended that the Belmont principles and related guidelines along with their interpretations do not adequately address *community*—a charge that he also levels at our version of principlism. Such a call for attention to community could mean, among other possibilities, that we should add community as a fifth principle or that we should interpret all principles in a communitarian rather than a merely individualistic frame. This second approach would involve reexamining the principles through the lens of community, and it is more promising. I see no justification for adding a separate principle of community; it does not appear to be necessary or helpful. However, I will note a few implications of using community as a lens for interpreting the four principles, especially in the context of research involving human subjects, the arena in which much of this discussion has occurred in recent years.

Beneficence already includes attention to the society's welfare, which has been part of the benefit to be balanced against the risks to subjects. However, attention to community might also require, as has become more frequent in discussions of nonmaleficence, attention to harms to particular communities, such as Native American communities, rather than merely harms to individuals.

Reinterpreted through the lens of community, the principle of respect for autonomy would consider persons not merely as isolated individuals, who consent or refuse to consent to participate in research, but also as members of communities. However, caution is also appropriate because it is not possible or justifiable to determine an individual's wishes and choices by reading them off community traditions, beliefs, and values, or to subordinate the individual's autonomy to the community's will.

Finally, justice concerns more than fairly selecting research subjects and fairly distributing the benefits and burdens of participating in research. It may include the participation of various communities in the design and evaluation of research. Beyond participation it might also include, for example, compensation for research-related injuries, as an expression of the community's solidarity with those who as research subjects assume a position of risk on behalf of the community and are non-negligently injured in the process. From this standpoint, it might not be sufficient to disclose on the consent form whether there will be any compensation for research-related injuries that are non-negligently caused; instead, compensation should be provided.

These examples suggest why it is important to revisit the principles again and again to make sure that their formulation and interpretation encompass the full range of relevant moral concerns. What is significant normatively about community can be incorporated through a more adequate interpretation of the four principles and derivative rules, without the addition of a separate principle.

Despite the claims of some proponents of a principle of community, *PBE* does not put primary weight on autonomy or *respect for* autonomy. We do not make autonomy the central value; indeed, the principle is respect for autonomy, not autonomy, and it is one prima facie principle along with others. It may often trump, but it does not have a priori superiority over, other principles. Indeed, I have argued sharply against overextending and overweighting the principle of respect for autonomy in relation to other general moral considerations (see Childress 1997a).

Perhaps several factors account for critics' misunderstanding of the place of respect for autonomy in *PBE*'s framework. One potential source of this misunderstanding is that we discuss respect for autonomy first among the four principles. However, it is important to distinguish (a) order of presentation of principles in a systematic examination, (b) order of consideration (e.g., in case analysis, which principle is considered first?), and (c) order of priority (which principle has the most weight or greatest strength?). The order of presentation, with the principle of respect for autonomy examined first in *PBE*, indicates nothing about the order of consideration, which will vary according to different kinds of real-life cases, or about the order of priority when principles and rules come into conflict. Again, respect for autonomy is simply one among equals, all prima facie binding.

Second, it is important to distinguish autonomy from respect for autonomy. In the first two editions, we contributed to a misinterpretation of our position by focusing on a "principle of autonomy" rather than a "principle of respect for autonomy." The former seems to impute a high value to personal autonomy and to indicate an ideal to which persons should aspire.

Third, I personally would interpret our framework as liberal communitarian. As noted earlier, it is communitarian in a methodological sense in that it focuses on the common morality. But, normatively speaking, in the context of public life, it is, I believe, *liberal* communitarian. In conflicts between the individual and the community, our framework stresses the presumptive, though nonabsolute, priority of respect for autonomy, including several rules derived from that principle, such as liberty and privacy, and requires that a significant, though not unreasonably heavy, burden of proof be discharged to justify coercive actions or policies. It is also liberal *communitarian* in its claims, for example, that social solidarity and communal beneficence, along with justice, require greater access to health care and fairer modes of allocation and distribution of health care.

PRINCIPLES AND CASES: SPECIFICATION AND CONSTRAINED BALANCING

Principles and Judgments about Cases

Some critics of *PBE*'s framework praise the book's "rich analysis" while rejecting the framework, as though the framework had little or nothing to do with the ethical analysis. For example, Ezekiel Emanuel comments that "one of the main reasons Beauchamp and Childress's analyses are so instructive is that they do not rigidly adhere to the very principles they elaborate" (Emanuel 1995, 38). He reports someone's comment that "the strength of Beauchamp and Childress's work was that in actual cases they did not practice what they preached." While I trust that these critics are correct that our analysis is rich, I believe that they have misunderstood our framework—it has never been as deductive as they suppose.

Unfortunately, our first edition included this sentence: "Moral judgments involve applications of action guides to concrete situations" (Beauchamp and Childress 1979, 6). We continued to use the language of "applied ethics" too long, and some of our charts gave the strong and wrong impression of a rigidly deductivist approach. But even in the first edition we approvingly quoted Joel Feinberg's point: "If a principle commits one to an antecedently unacceptable judgment, then one has to modify or supplement the principle in a way that does the least damage to the harmony of one's particular and general opinions taken as a group. On the other hand, when a solid well-entrenched principle entails a change in a particular judgment, the overriding claims of consistency may require that the judgment be adjusted." We then said: "The relations between the tiers of justification follow a similar dialectical pattern" (Beauchamp and Childress 1979, 12).

Indeed, in our initial proposal to Oxford, we wrote what I quoted earlier: "The principles are used throughout the book to help resolve moral problems that arise in the cases and the cases in turn are used as tests of the adequacy of the principles." That dialectical conception of the relation of principles and cases was present in the beginning and has remained throughout our work in progress, even if we emphasized it more strongly in some editions than in others and even though our heuristic charts sometimes misled people. We have struggled with how best to incorporate cases—a large number in the appendix or several incorporated into the text itself. I am not convinced that we have yet adequately addressed some of the key issues in case description along the lines that narrativists have raised.[1]

Now, as I have noted, not all moral judgments are—or should be— explicitly principle-based. Principles (and rules) primarily figure in moral reasoning when there is uncertainty and/or a conflict that needs to be resolved. Particular case judgments often proceed in relative independence of general moral principles or rules. We know what we ought to do and do it without reflecting on principles or rules, which we might articulate if someone asked us.

Sometimes principles may function even when they are not explicitly acknowledged or labeled. After the National Bioethics Advisory Commission had prepared its report *Cloning Human Beings* (NBAC 1997), one of the commissioners—a vocal critic of principlism—contended in conversation that "principles" had played no role in NBAC's deliberations about and recommendations for a ban, for three to five years, on human cloning. My response was that "NBAC's concern for safety reflects the principle of nonmaleficence and that NBAC at this time could not identify benefits of human cloning that outweigh the risk to children (a consideration of beneficence) or claims of autonomy in reproduction or in scientific inquiry strong enough to outweigh the risks to children. In addition, concerns about respect for persons, including their dignity as well as their autonomy, surfaced in discussions about objectifying and commodifying children. I would argue that these principles, and others, were transparent in NBAC's deliberations. . . . At the very least, the commission's consensus reflects its views about the respective weights of three prominent moral principles— nonmaleficence, beneficence, and respect for autonomy—in the context of recommending public policies regarding cloning" (Childress 1997b, 10). Furthermore, questions of justice also arose.

As *PBE* has evolved, we have tried to develop more clearly and in greater detail how our principles and rules relate to case judgments. Over a decade ago Henry Richardson (1990) helpfully analyzed and assessed three ways to connect principles/rules to concrete cases: deduction, balancing, and specification. If only one clear principle applies to an unambiguous factual situation, then deduction may be possible, but it is also likely to be uninteresting. Balancing and specification are more complex. *PBE* used both of them in earlier versions, but did not develop them very fully until the fourth edition in 1994, following the publication of Richardson's important essay.

Richardson's analytic framework is even more illuminating, I believe, when we distinguish two aspects or dimensions of moral principles and rules: (1) their range or scope of application; and (2) their weight, strength, or stringency. These aspects or dimensions are not totally independent, but are rather closely related, even when a particular framework makes one strategy primary for dealing with situations of conflict. Given these two dimensions, two basic questions emerge for various principlist approaches as they attempt to guide action.

Specification

One question is whether broad principles can be specified and concretized in more specific rules. Specification presupposes a distinction between general and specific and between degrees of generality and specificity. There is no hard and fast line between general and specific, since a moral species term may be a genus to some other term. However general our moral principles, we interpret them in part through more specific formulations or through the types of cases that fall under them. As R. M. Hare (1989, 54) notes, "any attempt to give content to a principle involves specifying the cases that are to fall under it. . . . Any principle, then, which has content goes some way down the path of specificity."

In addition, the distinction between principles and rules, which Richardson neglects in favor of the general term "norms," may be useful because rules are more specific than principles. And the distinction between the range or scope of applicability of a principle or rule, on the one hand, and its weight or strength, on the other hand, helps to clarify how specification works. Specification adjusts the circumstances of application of the relevant principles or rules, rather than adjusting their weight or strength relative to each other. Specification narrows the meaning, range, and scope of principles (and rules). For instance, the principle of respect for persons and their autonomous choices might be specified in a rule of informed consent or a rule of truthful disclosure to patients. As I noted earlier, *PBE* from the first edition on has engaged in such a process of specification, but we did not elaborate it as part of our method until Richardson's discussion (Richardson 1990, 2000). The fourth and fifth editions of *PBE* combine specification with constrained balancing.[2]

Specification is generally necessary and helpful, but it is also particularly appealing for absolutist positions because it provides a way to reduce conflicts between principles. An excellent example is the way the papal encyclical *Evangelium Vitae* starts from the biblical precept "you shall not kill" and indicates how the church moved to a more specific formulation in the context of difficult situations "in which values proposed by God's law seem to involve a genuine paradox." In seeking "a fuller and deeper understanding of what God's commandment prohibits and prescribes," the church developed more specific formulations that were consistent with the absolute and unchanging value of the commandment. The church's specification determined the precept's meaning by restricting its range and scope of application in at least two ways: first, to innocent persons, and, second, to direct actions (especially later in the process of specification). So the rule came to be interpreted as "Do not directly kill innocent persons" (Pope John Paul II 1994, Sec. 55, 57).

As a way to connect general principles to concrete cases, specification may still be subject to the charges of excessive appeals to intuition and arbitrariness that critics direct against efforts to balance moral norms (see Arras 1994). Furthermore, it may also involve balancing, as *PBE* emphasizes. Finally, I am also suspicious of absolutist approaches that seek to eliminate moral conflicts by specification.

Balancing Moral Principles

While specification focuses on the meaning, range, and scope of principles, a second question concerns how much weight, or what degree of stringency, different principles have, especially if they come into conflict in particular situations. If moral principles are more than merely advisory or illuminative, then it is important to determine just how binding they are in order to resolve conflicts that emerge.

Absolutism presents one extreme possibility: Absolutists might maintain that some moral principles and rules are absolutely binding whatever circumstances arise. But they could face irresolvable moral dilemmas if they recognize more than one absolute principle and those principles come into conflict. As a result, those who defend an absolutist position often carefully specify the meaning, range, and scope of their principles in order to avoid such conflicts (see Ramsey 1970; Pope John Paul II 1994; Childress 1996).

A second possible approach arranges principles in a lexical or serial order so that some principles must be satisfied before others can even be considered. In *A Theory of Medical Ethics*, for example, Robert Veatch (1981) assigns all deontological or nonconsequentialist principles, such as promise keeping, honesty, and not killing, "lexical priority over the principle of beneficence," a consequentialist principle. However, when deontological or nonconsequentialist principles themselves conflict, Veatch employs a "balancing strategy." Thus, while nonconsequentialist principles have "lexical ranking" over the principle of beneficence, they have "coequal ranking" in relation to each other. Such a lexical order breaks down in real-life situations, as do other absolutist approaches without considerable specification.

A third approach—our approach and perhaps the one most often associated with the term "principlism"—views moral principles as prima facie or presumptively binding, rather than as absolutely binding or lexically ordered. It thus balances these various principles when they come into conflict in particular cases. *PBE* holds that our four primary principles—respect for autonomy, nonmaleficence, beneficence (including utility or proportionality), and justice—along with such derivative rules as veracity, fidelity, privacy, and confidentiality—are all only prima facie binding. Thus, an act is morally right or obligatory insofar as it has the features that, according to the relevant principles, establish rightness or obligatoriness. For example, an act is right insofar as it is truthful, wrong insofar as it is a lie. However, a particular act, in particular circumstances, may have features that express some principles while contravening others—for instance, a truthful act may also cause harm or injustice. In such a case, the agent must determine whether one principle or the other is weightier or stronger, a judgment that cannot be made on the basis of prior, abstract formulations.

I have found this approach quite attractive for a long time—some version goes back to my work on W. D. Ross with William Christian, a philosopher of religion at Yale, and my dissertation, titled *Civil Disobedience and Political Obligation* (Childress 1971). Let me discuss prima facie obligations in relation to balancing and constraints on balancing.

What is the nature of a prima facie obligation or duty? (I use these terms interchangeably here even though it is useful to distinguish them in some settings.) W. D. Ross introduced the distinction between prima facie and actual obligations to account for conflicts of obligations, which, he maintained, proved to be "nonexistent" when fully and carefully analyzed (1930, 19–20). When two or more prima facie obligations come into conflict, we have to assess the total situation, including various possible courses of action with all their features of prima facie rightness and wrongness, to determine what we actually ought to do. The phrase "prima facie" indicates certain features of acts that have a tendency to make an act right or wrong and, thus, claim our attention; insofar as an act has those features it is right or wrong. But our actual obligation in the situation depends on the act in its wholeness and entirety. For "while an act may well be prima facie obligatory in respect of one character and prima facie forbidden in virtue of another, it becomes obligatory or forbidden only in virtue of the totality of its ethically relevant characteristics" (Ross 1939, 86). Prima facie does not mean "apparent" in contrast to "real," for prima facie duties are real even though they are distinguished from "actual" duties.

According to Ross, some prima facie obligations are more stringent than others (e.g., nonmaleficence, he claims, is more stringent than beneficence), and several duties (such as keeping promises) have "a great deal of stringency" (Ross 1930, 41–42). But he conceded that it is not possible to provide a complete ranking or a scale of stringency of obligations and quoted Aristotle: "The decision rests with perception" (Ross 1930, 42). Even though we intuit principles, according to Ross, we do not intuit what is right in the situation; rather we have to find "the greatest balance" of right over wrong. *PBE* does not engage in Ross's modest ranking or scaling (though I was tempted to take such an approach at one point)—all principles and rules are equally prima facie binding. We have to determine their actual weights in the situation.

So, to hold that an obligation or duty is prima facie is to claim that it always has a strong moral reason for its performance, but that this reason may not always, in every situation, be decisive or outweigh all other reasons. If an obligation is viewed as absolute, it cannot be overridden under any circumstances; it has priority over all other obligations with which it might conflict. If it is viewed as relative, the principle or rule stating that obligation amounts to a maxim or rule of thumb. It may illuminate but cannot prescribe what we ought to do. If it is construed as prima facie binding, it is intrinsically binding, but it does not necessarily determine one's actual obligation—that requires a balancing judgment in the situation, a judgment that is appropriately constrained by the kinds of questions posed in the next section.

An overridden or outweighed prima facie obligation continues to function in the situation and the course of action agents adopt. It leaves "moral traces" (to adopt a phrase from Robert Nozick 1968). It has or should have "residual effects" on the agent's actions and attitudes. As A. C. Ewing (1959, 110) suggests, "If I have a prima facie obligation which I cannot rightly fulfill because it is overruled by another, stronger prima facie obligation, it does not by any means follow that my conduct ought to be unaffected by the former obligation. Even if I am morally bound to do something inconsistent with it, it should in many cases modify in some respect the way in which the act is performed and in almost all it should affect some subsequent action." For example, if I think that a stronger obligation requires me to break a promise, I should at least explain the situation to the promisee, ask him not to hold me to the promise, apologize for breaking it, and even try to make it up to him later. At a minimum, Ewing (1959, 110) goes on to say, the prima facie obligation to keep the promise "should always affect our mental attitude toward the action" at least to the extent of evoking regret. According to W. D. Ross (1930, 28), "we do not for a moment cease to recognize a prima facie duty to keep our promise, and this leads us to feel, not indeed shame or repentance, but certainly compunction for behaving as we do." Specifiers lack that compunction. Nevertheless, legitimate debates persist about the attitudes and emotions agents should have both in deliberating about and in looking back at their actions that involved overriding one obligation in favor of another in a case of unavoidable conflict.

Constrained or Restricted Balancing of Prima Facie Principles

For critics, *PBE*'s form of principlism, which balances several prima facie principles, is excessively intuitive. In part to reduce the role of intuition, without denying it altogether, we have identified several conditions for "constrained balancing" (even though that characterization did not arise until the fifth edition). For instance, in the third edition (1989), we offered the following conditions for holding that one prima facie obligation overrides or outweighs another in particular circumstances:

1. The moral objective justifying the infringement must have a realistic prospect of achievement.
2. Infringement of a prima facie principle must be necessary in the circumstances, in the sense that there are no morally preferable alternative actions that could be substituted.
3. The form of infringement selected must constitute the least infringement possible, commensurate with achieving the primary goal of the action.
4. The agent must seek to minimize the effects of the infringement. (Beauchamp and Childress 1989, 53)

In the fifth edition (2001), in response to persistent criticisms that the model of balancing remains too intuitive and open-ended, we identified a longer list of conditions that restrict or constrain balancing:

1. Better reasons can be offered to act on the overriding norm than on the infringed norm. . . .
2. The moral objective justifying the infringement must have a realistic prospect of achievement.
3. The infringement is necessary in that no morally preferable alternative actions can be substituted.
4. The infringement selected must be the least possible infringement, commensurate with achieving the primary goal of the action.
5. The agent must seek to minimize any negative effects of the infringement.
6. The agent must act impartially in regard to all affected parties; that is, the agent's decision must not be influenced by morally irrelevant information about any party. (Beauchamp and Childress 2001, 19–20)

When these conditions are combined with requirements of coherence that we also insist on, they collectively provide a "reasonable measure of protection against purely intuitive or subjective judgments" (Beauchamp and Childress 2001, 21). Paraphrasing Aristotle, I would say that they provide us with as much precision as we can achieve given the subject matter of morality.

These conditions of constraint on intuition in balancing conflicting principles/rules are not new. Indeed, I recall that Sidney Hook once suggested that originality in moral, social, and political philosophy is almost always a sign of error. Similar (though more expansive) conditions have been elaborated in the just-war tradition. And I have argued that the just-war tradition can best be understood in terms of prima facie duties and constrained balancing.

In an article titled "Just-War Theories," which was published in *Theological Studies* in 1978, the year before the first edition of *PBE* appeared, I noted the similarities between the criteria that appear in the just-war tradition for the justification of the use of force and the criteria for justified civil disobedience, economic pressure, etc. (Childress 1978; see also Childress 1982). What accounts for these similarities? My contention was that we formulate and use criteria that are analogous to those featured in the just-war tradition whenever we face conflicting obligations or duties, one or more of which we cannot meet without infringing the other(s). In this sort of dilemma, we can justify infringing one obligation in order to meet another only when we can affirmatively answer certain questions. In effect, answering these questions serves to rebut the presumption against the use of lethal force, based on the principle of nonmaleficence. The language of "prima facie" suggests that there is a sufficient case for not using lethal force in the absence of justifying reasons that appeal to conflicting prima facie moral obligations or duties. Thus, we need to know whether we have a just cause, proper intentions, a reasonable hope of achieving the end, a reasonable balance between probable good and evil, and no other course of action that would enable us to realize the goal without sacrificing this obligation.

In short, the criteria for assessing wars and several other actions are similar because war and these other actions infringe some prima facie duties or obligations—an infringement that requires justification and can be justified along the lines suggested by the criteria. The use of force is only one of numerous human actions that stand in need of justification because they infringe prima facie obligations. There are others in biomedicine, and the framework of *PBE*, including its conditions of "constrained balancing," provides a way to address them.[3]

Conclusions: Into the Future

Despite various challenges, I still believe that *PBE* offers a helpful framework for moral discourse about biomedicine—it's not perfect, but I believe it is, overall, superior to its competitors. Some critics wonder whether, in view of the fact that the framework can be oversimplified or abused, it has been helpful on balance. I believe so, but obviously I am not a disinterested observer or assessor. Nevertheless, I recognize that *PBE* remains a work in progress—the metaphor I have emphasized in this essay—and that the framework it offers needs to be strengthened in various ways, in part by attending to what *PBE* neglects or downplays, sometimes because of space limitations but also because of focus, in part by addressing more adequately, through appropriate modifications, important criticisms, and in part by resolving some internal tensions in the framework.

Some of *PBE*'s omissions we coauthors deal with in our other scholarly lives. For instance, elsewhere (especially in *Practical Reasoning in Bioethics*, 1997a) I have dealt extensively with narrative, metaphor, and analogy, which are generally neglected in *PBE*. However, much remains to be done to integrate into our principlist framework the insights of various approaches to narrative on several levels, especially in case description. I would note, without developing the point here, that our version of principlism, which identifies several prima facie principles that must be interpreted and weighed in particular circumstances, may be more receptive to the insights of the narrativists than some forms of casuistry, especially forms that provide and require a tightly structured analysis of cases. Nevertheless, narrating cases involves issues that go beyond the analysis of principles and rules themselves, and these require further attention.

One major tension in our principlist framework, as I have suggested, concerns specification and constrained balancing in connecting principles and cases—Tom Beauchamp favors the former and I favor the latter, but we each, to some degree, recognize the necessity and value of the less-favored approach. A major challenge for us is to think through as carefully and imaginatively as possible how to conceive what I have called two aspects or dimensions of moral principles and rules—meaning, range, and scope, on the one hand, and weight, strength, or stringency, on the other. No conception of principles and rules and their application to or interpretation in particular situations can ignore either dimension—it is essential to consider both. And yet it is not easy to combine them in a coherent way. Another major challenge is to determine the exact nature and function of the constraints we propose on balancing.

Earlier I characterized *PBE*'s normative framework as liberal communitarian. Even though *PBE* has always and has increasingly attended to social and political philosophy—and not only moral philosophy—we need to develop our social and political philosophy more systematically, to show how the various principles and rules fit within a social and political perspective, and to indicate how social and political contexts partially shape presumptions, for instance, relating to respect for autonomy. In addition, I believe that the framework of *PBE* needs further elaboration and explication, beyond what we have provided to this point, for public deliberation in a democratic context. So much of what is critical in bio-ethics involves not only individual, familial, or professional decisions, but also the development of public policy. Even though the various editions of *PBE* recognize the centrality of public policy—defined, as one political theorist puts it, as "whatever governments do or do not do"—we need to develop more fully how our framework can function in public deliberation about public policy related to bioethics. And, in social philosophy, we need to address more adequately than we have the relation of the individual to various nongovernmental communities, such as the family and racial and ethnic groups.

Another area of political (and legal) philosophy that requires more attention than *PBE* has provided to date also relates to public deliberation. In certain conceptions of "public reason" in a liberal, pluralistic democratic polity, religious convictions about bioethics appear to be problematic, and yet many people ground their moral judgments about various bioethical issues in their religious convictions. No doubt religious convictions often flesh out interpretations of our four principles and related rules, for instance, by providing thick conceptions of goods and harms that are invoked in beneficence and nonmaleficence and by providing concrete rankings of principles and rules. But what is the appropriate role, if any, for religious convictions in the formation of public policy in contrast to the guidance of particular communities? And can principles and rules provide a framework for public deliberation without distorting and excluding thicker religious and nonreligious convictions? Sociologist John Evans's recent interpretation of the evolution of bioethics, particularly in relation to human genetic engineering, characterizes principlism as an effort to substitute formal rationality for substantive rationality in public bioethical debate and thereby to establish the legitimacy of bioethicists, over against theologians and the public (Evans 2002). This sociological interpretation is often provocative and sometimes illuminating, but it is problematic in various ways that will require sustained attention and response in another context.

Finally, I would like to develop and evaluate our framework of principles in international and global contexts, particularly in relation to the discourse about human rights. Even though I have not yet extensively pursued this topic, I believe that its exploration would be fruitful in so many ways, in part because *PBE*'s framework is familiar to many in other contexts and because they could offer important critiques from their standpoints. This conversation would help to clarify the possibilities and limits of "common morality," which, in any event, is not fully transparent and which requires discernment and interpretation.

NOTES

1. See, for example, Tod Chambers's various essays and *The Fiction of Bioethics* (1999).

2. See also DeGrazia 1992 for a defense of "specified principlism."

3. I am not the only one to draw connections between the just-war tradition and biomedical ethics—for instance, LeRoy Walters, whose doctoral dissertation focused on the just-war tradition, published in the late 1970s a splendid article on the parallels between the justification and limitation of research involving human subjects and the justification and limitation of war (Walters 1977).

REFERENCES

Arras, John. 1994. Principles and Particularity: The Roles of Cases in Bioethics. *Indiana Law Journal* 69: 983–1014.

Barad, Judith, with Ed Robertson. 2001. *The Ethics of Star Trek*. New York: Harper-Collins, Perennial Edition.

Beauchamp, Tom L., and James F. Childress. 1979. *Principles of Biomedical Ethics*. 1st ed. New York: Oxford University Press.

———. 1983. *Principles of Biomedical Ethics*. 2d ed. New York: Oxford University Press.

———. 1989. *Principles of Biomedical Ethics*. 3d ed. New York: Oxford University Press.

———. 1994. *Principles of Biomedical Ethics*. 4th ed. New York: Oxford University Press.

———. 2001. *Principles of Biomedical Ethics*. 5th ed. New York: Oxford University Press.

Brandt, Richard B. 1968. Toward a Credible Form of Utilitarianism. In *Contemporary Utilitarianism*, edited by Michael Bayles. Garden City, N.Y.: Doubleday Anchor Books.

———. 1979. *A Theory of the Good and the Right*. Oxford: Clarendon Press.

Chambers, Tod. 1999. *The Fiction of Bioethics: Cases as Literary Texts*. New York: Routledge.

Childress, James F. 1971. *Civil Disobedience and Political Obligation: A Study in Christian Social Ethics*. New Haven, Conn.: Yale University Press.

———. 1978. Just-War Theories: The Bases, Interrelations, Priorities, and Functions of Their Criteria. *Theological Studies* 39: 427–45.

———. 1982. *Moral Responsibility in Conflicts*. Baton Rouge: Louisiana State University Press.

———. 1996. Norms in Christian Ethics. In *Christian Ethics: Problems and Prospects*, edited by Lisa Sowle Cahill and James F. Childress. Cleveland: Pilgrim Press.

———. 1997a. *Practical Reasoning in Bioethics*. Bloomington: Indiana University Press.

———. 1997b. The Challenges of Public Ethics: Reflections on NBAC's Report. *Hastings Center Report* 27: 5, 9–11.

DeGrazia, David. 1992. Moving Forward in Bioethical Theory: Theories, Cases, and Specified Principlism. *Journal of Medicine and Philosophy* 17: 511–39.

Emanuel, Ezekiel J. 1995. The Beginning of the End of Principlism. *Hastings Center Report* 25 (July/August 1995): 37–38.

Evans, John H. 2002. *Playing God? Human Genetic Engineering and the Rationalization of Public Bioethical Debate*. Chicago: University of Chicago Press.

Ewing, A. C. 1959. *Second Thoughts in Moral Philosophy*. London: Routledge and Kegan Paul.

Frankena, William K. 1973. *Ethics*. 2d ed. Engelwood Cliffs, N.J.: Prentice Hall.

Hare, R. M. 1989. *Essays in Ethical Theory*. Oxford: Clarendon Press.

National Bioethics Advisory Commission (NBAC). 1997. *Cloning Human Beings*. Vol. I. Report and Recommendations of the National Bioethics Advisory Commission. Rockville, Md.: National Bioethics Advisory Commission.

Nozick, Robert. 1968. Moral Complications and Moral Structures. *Natural Law Forum* 13: 1–50.

Perlin, Seymour, ed. 1975. *A Handbook for the Study of Suicide*. New York: Oxford University Press.

Pope John Paul II. 1994. *Evangelium Vitae*. English Text. *Origins* 24, no. 42: 689–727.

Ramsey, Paul. 1970. *The Patient as Person*. New Haven, Conn.: Yale University Press.

Richardson, Henry S. 1990. Specifying Norms as a Way to Resolve Concrete Ethical Problems. *Philosophy and Public Affairs* 19: 279–310.

———. 2000. Specifying, Balancing, and Interpreting Bioethical Principles. *Journal of Medicine and Philosophy* 25: 285–307.

Ross, W. D. 1930. *The Right and the Good*. Oxford: Clarendon Press.

———. 1939. *Foundations of Ethics*. Oxford: Clarendon Press.

Veatch, Robert M. 1981. *A Theory of Medical Ethics*. New York: Basic Books.

Walters, LeRoy. 1977. Some Ethical Issues in Research Involving Human Subjects. *Perspectives in Biology and Medicine* (winter 1977): 193–211.

4

Revisiting *A Theory of Medical Ethics*: Main Themes and Anticipated Changes

ROBERT M. VEATCH

I n the mid-1960s, when I chose to devote my career to the study of biomedical ethics, there was no such thing as a formal theory of medical ethics. There were, of course, bits and pieces of theory— the Hippocratic oath and the American Medical Association (AMA) Code of Ethics in professional medicine; various theologically based stances about medical morality; and some volumes by secular and religious authors on specific topics in medical ethics. It rapidly became clear to me that doing medical ethics from various religious or secular ethical traditions would produce radically different answers to moral dilemmas than those that could be derived from the fragments of theory available within the health care professions.

THE HISTORY

When I completed graduate school and joined Dan Callahan and Will Gaylin as the first member of the staff of the Institute of Society, Ethics and the Life Sciences (The Hastings Center), my first assignment was to coordinate the development of a medical ethics teaching program at Columbia University's College of Physicians and Surgeons. I quickly became frustrated with the topically oriented quandary approach to medical ethics in which someone presented a case dilemma about what to tell a dying patient or whether to spend resources dialyzing a man whose social support network suggested the therapy would fail. I began seeking some more systematic way of thinking about problems in medical ethics, a search that eventually led me to write *A Theory of Medical Ethics* (1981). Since I am currently beginning a long-term project to completely revise the book and produce a new edition, I will take this opportunity to sketch the kinds of themes and ideas that will be more fully developed in that edition.

My first effort in the direction of systematizing medical ethics was to attempt to collect and organize more methodically the cases we encountered on the hospital floor and in many clinical consultations. That led to the volume *Case Studies in Medical Ethics* (Veatch 1977). That, however, did not accomplish all of what I had in mind—a systematic account of a theoretical framework by which one could consistently approach any issue in the ethics of medicine or health care.[1] By the mid-1970s I had completed the first of my case book series[2] as well as the first edition of my examination of the ethics of terminal care, *Death, Dying, and the Biological Revolution* (1976). I now had the opportunity to begin a project that had been on my mind for some time: the construction of an overall, systematic theory of medical ethics. This work was carried on alongside my normal work at the Hastings Center, which was to administer the Center's Death and Dying Research Group, as well as its Health Policy Research Group.

By systematic theory I mean an account that starts with the most fundamental metaethical questions: What is the meaning of ethical terms? What is the ultimate foundation of ethical norms? And how do humans know what those norms are? The account would then move on to matters of normative theory: a theory of value (axiology); a theory of morally right action (including a set of principles or other moral norms) that provides a small set of very abstract morally right-making criteria of behavior; and perhaps a set of virtues as well.

These first two stages would surely constitute the major part of a systematic theory of medical ethics, but would not be the entire story. We would also have to include an account of how one might move from the level of normative ethical theory with its values and principles and virtues, to the individual case decision, whether that decision is made in the clinic, in the courts, or in the privacy of the patient's home without the benefit of professional assistance. We might need a set of rules or rights to mediate between the abstract principles and the individual decision. We would at least need an account of what role, if any, a code of moral rules or rights should play in that process.

By the mid-1970s I was aware that the goal of a systematic account of a medical ethical theory was worth pursuing. What I have described we would now call a "top down" approach to theory. As a student of

John Rawls at Harvard, I was already familiar with the concept of *reflective equilibrium* and had no reservations about working both up and down this hierarchy of theory elements, what I now call the "ladder of levels of medical ethics." A full diagram of this "ladder" appears on the inside cover of the second edition of *The Basics of Bioethics* (2003).

By 1979 I had prepared first drafts of most of the major sections of *A Theory of Medical Ethics.* That year Tom Beauchamp and Jim Childress published the first edition of their *Principles of Biomedical Ethics* (1979), which, while it eschewed discussion of metaethics, presented a coherent and widely adopted analysis of a principle-based approach to medical ethics.[3] I was able to adjust my manuscript to some extent in the final draft to take their first edition into account. In December of that year, I moved from the Hastings Center to the Kennedy Institute of Ethics, a move that gave me the luxury of time as well as talented research support that made it possible to complete the manuscript.

THE CONCEPTUAL ISSUES: FIVE MAJOR THEMES

The construction of the theory begins with an account in the first three chapters of the radically different medical ethical systems existing in the world. What is most critical for purposes of medical ethical theory is that almost all of these theories exist completely outside organized professional medicine. They are not grounded in any "internal morality of medicine" or any moral perspective from within the medical professions. The *Ethical and Religious Directives for Catholic Health Facilities* (United States Catholic Conference 1971; cf. later editions including National Conference of Catholic Bishops 2001), for example, bases the medical ethics that can be gleaned from the long list of codified rules on the metaethics of Roman Catholic moral theology, on its theory of the role of reason, revelation, church tradition, and papal authority in knowing what is moral. Transferring this metaethic that is in its foundations external to medicine into the field of health care would make sense for Roman Catholic doctors and patients, but would not be appropriate for Jewish, Hindu, or secular people. I have recently developed further the theme of these first three chapters: that all medical ethics must have its metaethical foundations outside of medicine (Veatch 2001).

Looking back on *A Theory of Medical Ethics*, I can identify five major themes that I think constitute the book's unique contribution. I will outline those before turning to five lingering problems.

1. The Death of the Hippocratic Ethic

The first breakthrough in my own mind was the eventual realization that the old Hippocratic oath was a terribly implausible, indeed immoral basis for practicing almost any kind of medicine that people in any culture of the world would accept. Its core principle, that the physician should work always to benefit the patient and to protect the patient from harm, offends any believer in the Universal Declaration of Human Rights because it recognizes no such rights. It offends Kantians because it has no universalizable maxims independent of patient benefit. It offends all who subscribe to liberal political philosophy because it is blatantly paternalistic and lacks any principle of patient autonomy. It offends social utilitarians because it requires excluding consideration of all benefits other than the patient's. It offends anyone who is Jewish or Christian or Marxist because it has no concept of social justice. It offends Muslims, Hindus, Confucians, and those who subscribe to various African tribal religions. In *Theory* I summarize these major offenses by characterizing the Hippocratic oath as individualistic, consequentialistic, and paternalistic, a combination that virtually no moral tradition anywhere in the world should find acceptable. The first and perhaps most important contribution of *Theory* was to show that no rational person—patient or provider—living today could possibly accept the Hippocratic tradition. It may have worked for that group of Greek physicians in the fourth century B.C.E. who subscribed to what was apparently a Pythagorean mystery cult, but not for any modern human being and not for almost all humans of the ancient world, such as Jews and Christians.[4] The first theme of *Theory* was that there are many "proto-theories" or incipient theories of medical ethics in the world and that all of them have some important differences from the Hippocratic tradition.

2. The Triple Contract

I set out in chapter 4 of *Theory* to examine the problems with the meta-ethics of traditional professional ethics and in chapter 5 to begin the construction of an alternative metaethics that could be adapted to both religious and secular ethical systems. The result was what I called a "triple contract theory." Three major influences shaped that development. First, I came to medical ethics from a background in research neuropharmacology. I began my career as an empirical medical scientist. As such I had empiricist inclinations. Second, I was, at Harvard, a student of John Rawls and was introduced to his version of contract theory when *A Theory of Justice* was read in manuscript by his students.[5] Third, I was a product of the branch of the Judeo-Christian tradition that was both covenantal and empiricist. Judeo-Christian reliance on covenant as a way of describing sets of moral norms is, in my view, nothing more than a branch of, indeed the original model for, social contract theory. While this suggestion has led Bill May (1975) to be concerned that the differences between religious covenant and secular contract are not being maintained adequately, I continue to insist that the classical secular contract theorists (Locke, Hobbes, Rousseau, and the American founding fathers) are the descendants of Judeo-Christian covenant doctrine. It is not an accident, for example, that the modern Protestant theologian John Wesley was a student of John Locke and the empiricist tradition.

The First Contract

Thus, my metaethical theory begins with the societal responsibility of articulating a basic set of ethical principles (together with, perhaps, human rights as well as virtues). I follow Rawls and the ancient Hebrew tradition in holding that the moral norms can best be articulated by imagining human beings gathering together to attempt to agree on a set of basic ethical truths. It is not unlike the gathering of the Israelites after the exile to articulate the community's norms (Nehemiah 10:28–31). Just like the Israelites, we should imagine all manner of people at such a gathering. This, as James Madison knew, would tend to neutralize idiosyncratic biases and approximate what reason requires. If the goal is a set of *moral* norms rather than a mere political compromise, everyone at the table should strive to be as objective as possible—as if they were blinded to their own special values, interests, and knowledge limits. They should, in short, strive to be like ideal scientists attempting to discover and articulate a truth about the universe.

The only difference between these contractors and those attending an international scientific meeting is the subject matter they are attempting to describe. Since any real-life effort at social contracting to articulate the basic norms is limited by the finitude and fallibility of humans, we know that any actual human effort will be less than perfect. However, we can claim that, hypothetically, if the social contractors were perfect observers—ideal observers, to use Roderick Firth's term (1952)—their product would be an agreed-upon set of moral norms that is at least one of the perfect accounts of a moral system.[6] Thus, if it is believed that there is a set of universal moral norms existing in the universe, this first, hypothetical social contract (or covenant) would articulate the principles (and perhaps the rights, rules, and virtues) that describe those norms. That is merely what we *mean* when we say that there is a set of universal ethical norms.

The Second Contract

Assuming this first, hypothetical contract is established, we can then move on to explore a second set of norms governing the relation between medical lay people and medical professionals—nurses, pharmacists, physicians, and so forth. My "second contract" is one between the general public and members of the medical professions considered collectively. One can think of it as an idealized version of the negotiation between the public and the professions to establish the conditions of licensure. The result of that negotiation is, in fact, a set of conditions for lay and professional behavior that lead to a mutual agreement or "contract" between the parties. This contract might, for instance, authorize physicians to violate normal rules of invasion of bodily privacy, specify limits on physician behavior (such as the Tarasoff rule for confidentiality), and impose duties on lay people in the lay-professional relation. Carol Spicer and I (Veatch and Spicer 1992; Veatch and Spicer 1993; Veatch 1994) have more recently argued that the duty of the physician to deliver certain treatments desired by patients or surrogates that violate the conscience of the physician (so-called "futile care") is a duty that derives from this contract of licensure between provider and public. Even though ordinary citizens have rights grounded in the principle of autonomy that permit them to refuse to deliver such services that violate conscience, physicians may be bound by this second contract, under the principle of fidelity to promises, to provide certain treatments.

Likewise, the second contract presently imposes on physicians, nurses, and other health professionals certain other constraints: not to kill for mercy; not to prescribe the use of heroin, even for patients who could benefit from it; and not to touch a patient without an adequately informed consent.

As with the first contract, the terms of this second contract may not be expressed perfectly at the present time. It is theoretically possible, for example, that the traditional prohibition on physician killing for mercy is not what hypothetical ideal observers of the medical relationship would endorse. There always remains the possibility that the actual contract is erroneous as long as the real-life contractors are finite and fallible. We know this is true because not all cultures understand the duty of people in the professional role in the same way. At least some of them are undoubtedly somewhat mistaken. The point of this model, however, is that the correct norms for the lay-professional relationship are the ones that hypothetical ideal contractors—lay people and professional—would agree to. They are not a product that the profession, by itself, invents or even discovers. Nor are they the product of the lay population. Needless to say, that means they are not the product of any real-life government agency or professional organization. They are the norms that hypothetical, ideal contractors in lay and professional roles would agree to. Hence, any effort by a professional organization to formulate moral norms unilaterally, such as the World Medical Association's recent effort with regard to norms for research on human subjects, is a mistaken methodology (even if it were to turn out that this document produced a reasonable approximation of the proper norms). Most citizens of the moral community are excluded from membership in the organizations at the table to produce the revised declaration. The result is likely to be a distortion. Subjects are woefully underrepresented; researchers terribly overrepresented.

When we turn to this second contract, those in a liberal society are likely to believe that the norms of the original social contract might give some space for some options in specifying the norms of the various lay and professional roles. This could mean, for example, that the parties of the second contract, in addition to being bound by the norms of the first contract and any requirements of hypothetical contractors at the second level, may also be able to invent some actual norms for health professionals and lay people that are not necessarily required by the hypothetical reflections (but are not prohibited by them either). This means there will be space for individual cultures to add some specific, actual norms as long as they do not violate any of the universal norms from the first or second contracts.

I view the prohibition on prescribing heroin in this regard. I am convinced that neither the first contract nor the hypothetical requirements of the second contract *require* a prohibition on heroin prescribing. Those countries that permit it are thus, it seems to me, within their rights—indeed, I suggest morally wise, because they give adequate space to meet the needs of those suffering most severely—as required by the prima facie principle of justice. However, it may be that a society and its professionals could also agree to ban this practice of heroin use. Thus the terms of the hypothetical second contract are sometimes permissive. They permit some actual contractual limits on lay and professional roles without requiring those limits. In the United States, for example, we presently permit both fee-for-service private practice and the common, more socialized forms of practice, whether in managed care, capitation payments, and government programs such as Medicare, Medicaid, the VA, and the Civilian Health and Medical Program for the Uniformed Services (CHAMPUS). Even if some current American health care policy is so offensive that it violates the norms of any appropriate lay-professional relations, some elements of private, fee-for-service medicine are probably morally tolerable.

The Third Contract: The Individual Lay-Professional Contract

Just as the first contract left space for society to create a second contract establishing lay and professional roles that have some variability, so the second contract seems to leave a great deal of space for lay people and professionals to negotiate individual agreements establishing the goals and limits of their relationship. This third contract is the one that permits both lay people and professionals to agree on certain limits to their interactions. A patient and surgeon may (but need not) agree to ban forgoing resuscitation while in the operating room. Lay people and professionals may agree to either more palliative or more cure-oriented terminal care without violating any fundamental moral norms.

When we get to the level of this third—more individual—contract, I assume that we are dealing primarily, maybe exclusively, with an actual contract, one that operates within the spaces created by the liberties of the first and second contracts.

It is this third contract that many critics seem to have in their sights when they take potshots at contract theory. They attack contract theory as being too individualistic, too legalistic, and too business-like. That charge may be appropriate for certain contract theories of medical ethics that limit contract theory to actual individual relations—to some primitive Engelhardtian liberal contract, for example. It surely does not apply to the kind of hypothetical, three-stage social contract I propose here, one that is grounded in Judeo-Christian and secular social contract theory that is, at its core, societal, philosophical, and normative; not individualistic, legalistic, and businesslike.

3. Going beyond Patient Welfare: Duty-based Principles at the Individual Level

The third major element of *A Theory of Medical Ethics* is its movement beyond Hippocratic patient welfare. I claim that the effect of the triple contract would be to recognize that the norms of society and those of the lay-professional relation require going beyond patient benefit and protection of the patient from harm. That movement, I suggested in

Theory, must come in two different directions: (1) by adding principles imposing moral duty on our individual patient-provider relations beyond benefit and harm, and (2) by embedding these norms in a set of social ethical principles.

The first set of additional norms I referred to as "deontological" or duty-based. These norms share the feature that they describe right-making characteristics of actions that are independent of consequences. They include the principle of autonomy (or respect for autonomy) that has been present in Beauchamp and Childress (1979, 56–96) from their first edition. It has been present in both modern Protestant and secular Kantian ethical systems. It imposes severe limits on the physician's right (and therefore his or her duty) to benefit and protect the patient from harm. In contrast with Beauchamp and Childress, however, *Theory* includes other Kantian/Protestant principles: principles that I called *contract keeping, honesty*, and *avoiding killing* (and I now usually call *fidelity, veracity*, and *avoiding killing*).

In contrast with others working in this area of theory construction, I see these as independent moral norms that cannot be derived from or reduced to respect for autonomy (Beauchamp and Childress 2001), permission (Engelhardt 1996), or nonmaleficence (Gert, Culver, and Clouser 1997). To see the implication, my position holds that there are obligations to keep promises to individuals who are not and never can be autonomous agents. One likewise must fulfill (prima facie) the obligations of veracity to nonautonomous persons and cannot kill people even if the killing is unrelated to the loss of their autonomy (cf. Beauchamp and Childress 2001; Engelhardt 1996). Likewise, one cannot break a promise, violate autonomy, or kill just because doing so would in a particular case not cause harm (cf. Gert, Culver, and Clouser 1997).

The inclusion of a principle of avoiding killing is unusual in modern philosophical ethical systems, but commonplace in more traditional ethics. The idea here is that the prohibition on killing cannot be reduced to cases in which people will be harmed if they are killed or to those in which people will lose their autonomy if they are killed. There is something prima facie morally wrong-making about killing someone who is a living human being (and perhaps also some who are living nonhumans).

The result is that I proposed a cluster of four principles that challenge the Hippocratic ethic and impose severe limits on the right of health professionals to benefit patients. They cannot benefit patients by violating their autonomy, by breaking promises to them, by telling them lies, or by mercifully killing them—or, at least, doing any of these things would violate these norms that are not grounded in production of good consequences.

4. Going beyond Patient Welfare: The Social Ethical Principles

The second set of additional norms moves the focus to the social level. The consequence-maximizing principles of beneficence and nonmaleficence— which I sometimes combine to call a principle of utility—apply not only to patient welfare, but also to other parties and to society as a whole. If consequences are limited to patient welfare, virtually all human-subjects research, all public health, and all cost-containment efforts become immoral, yet almost all rational persons accept the importance of these activities at least in some cases. Likewise, I included another ethical principle at the social level that is parallel to the deontological or duty-based principles at the level of the individual. Just as autonomy or fidelity or veracity or avoiding killing may impose limits on the right of clinicians to benefit the individual patient, so the principle of *justice* imposes limits on the principles of beneficence and nonmaleficence at the social level. In *Theory*, justice was a principle that potentially conflicts not only with Hippocratic utility, but also social utility.

5. Ranking and Balancing Conflicting Principles

The fifth conceptual development in *Theory* that I wish to highlight is confronting the probability that any medical ethical theory is likely to incorporate more than one ethical principle. Even various forms of the now-discredited Hippocratic ethic must address how beneficence is related to nonmaleficence. Is it to consider benefits and harms by subtracting expected patient harms from the benefits; to calculate the ratio of benefits to harms; or to follow the non-Hippocratic slogan "first of all do no harm," meaning that prevention of harm is given a special priority in the moral calculus? When more principles are added, as occurs in most sophisticated normative ethical theories beyond Hippocratism, the problem of conflict among principles becomes more complex.

In *Theory*, I developed a unique answer to the question of how conflicts among principles should be resolved. I began with the observation that in the contemporary informed consent debate, at least in the United States, the autonomy of the competent patient *always* takes precedence over the physician's desire to benefit the patient. That at least is our well-considered moral judgment. This seems to me, on reflection, to be right. That means that any theory of resolving conflict among principles cannot balance competing claims between patient welfare and patient autonomy. It must give priority to autonomy. Likewise, I am convinced that the considered moral judgment is that, at least in normal cases, it is unacceptable to violate the truth-telling principle merely to benefit a competent patient paternalistically. In the same vein, it is unacceptable to break a promise just to benefit the patient. Something more is needed, such as patient permission to lie, break promises, or violate autonomy (in which case arguably what remains is no longer a lie, a broken promise, or an autonomy violation).

On the other hand, I know of no way to rank-order the four principles that I have classified as nonconsequentialist: fidelity, autonomy, veracity, and avoiding killing. When these conflict among themselves, I know of no alternative but to balance the competing claims. Only when the duty-based (perfect) duties are satisfied can one strive to benefit the patient. It is also plausible that, if there are ties among the duty-based principles, net patient welfare should be the tie-breaker.

At the social level, it is less obvious that the duty-based (nonconsequentialist) principles should similarly take absolute precedence. Nevertheless, I argued in *Theory* that that should be the case. One might be skeptical of this conclusion because it seems obvious, for example, that in some cases public health concerns should justify constraints on autonomy even though that would seem to mean that social utility is overriding autonomy. Opening the door to permitting social utility to trump rights grounded in autonomy and other duty-based principles could, however, be both dangerous and counterintuitive. It would permit any degree of harm to an unconsenting human subject, for example, provided only that the social benefit were great enough. What is needed is a limited basis for overriding autonomy without opening the floodgates so that it is swamped in a sea of social utility.

I think that comes by permitting violation of autonomy when, and only when, some other duty-based principle competes with autonomy. This would mean that previous promises made, the need to avoid killing, or the need to promote justice could all justify overriding autonomy even though merely promoting good consequences could not. Thus, the needs of persons at risk for being worst off could justify violating autonomy but not social benefits to the well-off. It is not the amount of benefit, but who benefits that counts morally as a justification for overriding autonomy. The result would be a cautious basis for limited overriding of autonomy without subordinating it to considerations of aggregate utility. Likewise, this approach would logically open the door to very limited breach of the principle of avoiding killing, but only in the name of acting justly toward those who are among the worst off, never in the name of mere production of increased social utility. Since killing of competent and formerly competent people against their will always violates autonomy, this limited justice-based opening to mercy killing would probably only be tolerable when it does not violate autonomy. That surely is the kind of reasoning that Paul Ramsey had in mind when he admitted very limited exceptions to the principle of avoiding killing (Ramsey 1970, 161–64).

This approach has the quality of giving the duty to avoid lying, breaking promises, killing, and so forth a moral priority over producing benefits in a way that superficially resembles the position of Gert, Culver, and Clouser (1997, 5, 7, 21, 76), but I reject their claim that these are rules derived from the not-harming principle, which is the only principle that they take as morally obligatory.

THE CURRENT RELEVANCE

I have found these five basic conceptual themes remarkably stable and consistent with a very wide range of considered moral judgments. The new edition of *Theory* is likely to retain most of these elements. Related to these, however, is a set of current problems in medical ethical theory that needs more attention.

In the years since *Theory* first appeared, much has happened in medical ethics. The advances in medical technology—stem cell research, transplant rejection protocols, and rationing strategies—have been paralleled by advances in medical ethical theory. Since I wrote the first edition of *Theory*, four more editions of the *Principles of Biomedical Ethics* have appeared. To these we can add two editions of Tristram Engelhardt's *Foundations of Bioethics* (1986 and 1996); Baruch Brody's *Life and Death Decision Making* (1988); Ed Pellegrino and David Thomasma's *For the Patient's Good* (1988); and Bernie Gert, Chuck Culver, and Danner Clouser's *Bioethics: A Return to Fundamentals* (1997). These are all general statements of systematic approaches to medical ethics that could plausibly be called medical ethical theories. (They are, in fact, the books I teach in my graduate-level course titled "Theories of Medical Ethics.") The newly planned edition of *Theory* will be much harder to write because I now have these sophisticated alternatives to consider. I will no doubt steal many good ideas, but I will also undoubtedly refrain from adopting many others. Five areas need attention in the light of more recent developments.

1. Common Morality and the Triple Contract

Both the new edition (2001) of Beauchamp and Childress and the recent Gert, Culver, and Clouser (1997) ground medical ethical theory in something they call the common morality. This is largely an empirical claim—that as a matter of fact "everyone" (Gert, Culver, and Clouser 1997, 1) or all "morally serious" (Beauchamp and Childless 2001, 3) people of the world accept certain norms as morally authoritative. Since it seems quite obvious that not literally "everyone" accepts this morality, the concept requires some limiting phrase such as "virtually everyone," "all reasonable people," or all "morally serious people." Of course, these limiting phrases might be self-fulfilling since one might label anyone who does not accept the core common morality as "unreasonable" or "not serious." The question to be addressed is whether this empirical claim can be connected to the metaethical claim that there exists a single universal core set of moral norms—or, at least, that such a set should be spoken of as if it existed in reality. The fact that there was universal agreement would not necessarily impress if the moral norms agreed to turn out to be wrong. Flat earth theory, magically caused illness, and justified slavery all come to mind as areas about which very widespread agreement now appears to have been wrong. On the other hand, for those who believe that a single universal set of moral norms should be treated as if it existed in reality, the empirical finding that there is a common morality might not be surprising.

I am, in general, sympathetic with the claim that there is a common morality—as an empirical and as a metaethical claim. As one originally trained in the empirical natural sciences, however, I am left with the necessary qualifier that, no matter how confident someone is of an empirical claim and how unanimous the agreement, the existing consensus may be mistaken. I am inclined to be somewhat more of a scientific skeptic. I am convinced that all human observers (short of the hypothetical ideal observer) are fallible. They are likely, especially at the margins, to make mistakes. More critically, the generalities subsumed under the heading of "common morality" may mask more subtle differences across cultures. The "principle of avoiding killing," as I used it, does not mean exactly the same thing as the widely shared "principle of the sacredness of life" or the Jewish notion that all human life should be preserved. I insist on the distinction between the set of principles that hypothetical ideal observers would commit to and those that real-world, finite people actually accept as a morality held in common by all people of the world. When one adds to this the agreed-upon observation that the specific applications of the generalities of the common morality will necessarily be contingent on the facts of the situation, we can remain confident that there is a more or less common morality among at least most morally serious people and that the odds seem good that these people get that morality more or less right.

2. Beneficence, Nonmaleficence, and Pellegrino

I have already mentioned that, even for the traditional Hippocratic medical ethic, there is considerable controversy over how estimates of benefit and harm should be combined. Should harms be subtracted from benefits? Should ratios be calculated? Or should not harming get priority, as Gert, Culver, and Clouser and the *primum non nocere* advocates suggest?

The addition of benefits and harms to other parties—that is, of social consequentialism—to the Hippocratic ethic makes matters much more complicated. For about two centuries, organized medicine, from Thomas Percival to the most recent codes of the AMA, has been struggling with the problem of how to correct the obvious Hippocratic error of claiming that the physician's only duty is to benefit the patient. That would mean physicians have a moral duty to ignore their spouses and children whenever a patient could be helped. That would mean that physicians have a duty to ignore all their own welfare in violation of Rossian duties of self-improvement.[7] It would mean physicians have a duty to ignore research medicine, public health, and cost containment (except in those special cases where these activities will benefit the physician's patient).

Percival began to speak of duties of the physician to society. The AMA code of 1847 continued that correction, as have all the codes since then. Only in 2001 has the AMA begun to imply that perhaps this trend has gone too far. It amended its code to call to its members' attention that the primary duty of the physician is to the individual patient (AMA 2001).

My problem is even greater than the AMA's. I must not only reexamine whether my proposal to balance net benefits to the patient against net benefits to society with each counting equally can be defended, but also reexamine the strategy of subordinating all consideration of benefit and harm to any of the other principles. I must also deal with Ed Pellegrino's idiosyncratic claim that autonomy can never conflict with beneficence because patient autonomy is not only one of the elements in his theory of the good but also an element that ranks higher than the medical good (Pellegrino and Thomasma 1988, 156, 159). That means that promoting the patient's good seems to always require respecting patient autonomy when it conflicts with the patient's medical good.

I think that Pellegrino must be mistaken here. It is true that his theory might always require respecting autonomy when autonomy theorists believe it should be respected. But it faces other problems. For one, Pellegrino's concept of the good for the patient includes four levels: the patient's biomedical good, the patient's concept of his own good, the good of the patient as a person, and the ultimate good. The autonomy of the patient thus takes precedence over the patient's medical good, but at the same time the ultimate good and the patient's concept of his or her own good (patient autonomy) are both higher in ranking than the autonomy of the patient and should supersede the patient's autonomously chosen preference. Autonomy ought to lose sometimes under the Pellegrino theory of the good.

Second, even if his theory recognizes patient autonomy as prevailing in exactly the right cases, it misses the underlying reason why patient choice should be respected. Those who are committed to the normative principle of autonomy do not favor it simply because it promotes the patient's good; if so, they would abandon autonomy whenever the patient's good would be served (as in when a higher-order good takes precedence). They favor autonomy because it is an independent right-making characteristic of action. Pellegrino and other teleologists (including Thomist teleologists) reject this claim, but for deontologists (including Kantians, rights theorists, those who subscribe to liberal political philosophy, Protestants, Jews, and others with deontological inclinations) the distinction between respecting a patient's autonomy and promoting a patient's good is critical.

3. Avoiding Killing: Its Relevance for Euthanasia

A third area needing additional work involves my interpretation of the principle of avoiding killing. I interpreted it as holding that active killing of a human is a wrong-making characteristic of actions. I argued that it did not apply in the same fashion to omissions of life support. I explicitly relied on the omission/commission distinction rather than the intention/foreknowledge distinction, which I held was relevant to evaluating character, but not the morality of actions.

It is clear that active killing for mercy is more open for discussion today than it was in 1981. Recent commentators in the debate either continue to apply the double effect doctrine (i.e., the intention/foreknowledge distinction: Pellegrino and Thomasma 1988, 204, 206) or they reduce the ethics of killing to the ethics of avoiding harm (Gert, Culver, and Clouser 1997, 76; Beauchamp and Childress 2001, 117, 141–42). It is clear that killing people usually harms them and the principle of nonmaleficence is usually sufficient to explain why it is morally wrong to kill (as, incidentally, is the principle of autonomy). But the interesting case has become the one in which someone is not harmed by killing and, in fact, the killing can be seen as preventing future harms.

My approach to avoiding killing walks a delicate intermediate course. Killing humans is always prima facie wrong, *and* beneficence and nonmaleficence alone cannot overcome that wrongness. Consequence-maximizing principles cannot justify overriding duties that are independent of consequences. In fact, if beneficence and nonmaleficence could override the principle of avoiding killing, that would justify killing off any people who burden society so much that keeping them alive is a greater harm than the harm done to the individual if he is killed.[8]

My unique way of balancing competing moral claims permits other principles to be balanced against avoiding killing even though the utility-maximizing principles cannot be. For example, respect for autonomy might counterbalance avoiding killing, at least to the point of leaving one morally perplexed about the ethics of rational suicide. More critically, even if the utility-maximizing principles cannot counterbalance avoiding killing, perhaps justice can. This would mean that determining whether the patient is among the worst off in his or her suffering is morally relevant in deciding whether a rare exception must be made to the prima facie principle that requires avoiding killing. The result would be that the overwhelming presumption is against killing and that mere beneficence and nonmaleficence cannot overcome that presumption. Since the principle of autonomy can be relevant in counterbalancing the principle of avoiding killing, one should be more inclined to treat merciful killing as tolerable if it is substantially autonomous—that is, if it is a rational suicide. Nevertheless, one could imagine an extreme case in which justice alone would offset avoiding killing if the incompetent patient were suffering so overwhelmingly as to place the individual among those with the strongest claims of justice.[9] The result is a strong presumption against active merciful killing, one that cannot be overcome by mere consideration of benefit and harm but can potentially be overcome by extreme claims of justice, especially if the principle of autonomy also weighs in on that side. If I can sustain the claim of the first edition of *Theory* that the principle of avoiding killing extends only to actions and not to omissions, then I end up with a position that need not rely on the charade of the double effect doctrine to explain every forgoing of treatment, even those that seem boldly to be for the purpose of letting death occur rather than merely forgoing some useless or burdensome intervention.

4. Justice

The introduction of the principle of justice suggests a fourth area that needs further attention in the light of the current state of scholarship. I have made several previous attempts to articulate my theory of the principle of justice as an egalitarian one, one that supports equality of opportunities to be as healthy as other people. Some have labeled this an extreme or radical egalitarian view, perhaps failing to grasp that I treat all principles, including the principle of justice, as prima facie. Just as one can accept the principle of autonomy as requiring complete respect for individual choices grounded in autonomously chosen life-plans without committing to the inevitable dominance of autonomy when it conflicts with other (duty-based) principles, so also one can accept the principle of justice as requiring opportunities for equality of well-being without committing to the inevitable dominance of justice when it competes with other principles.

I have, especially in earlier work, tended to treat health care as morally special, not because it is more important or prior to other goods, but because need for health care is radically unequal. If we provide equal access to a generalized medium such as money, we can rely on approximately equal need for food, clothing, shelter, etc., to produce fair equality of opportunity, since the need for these is more or less equally distributed. If one person chooses to spend a larger proportion of resources on food and another on shelter, we should not be concerned about inequities.[10] Health care (along with education) is unique. If people given an equal amount of some generalized medium such as money have to spend some portion of their resources on health care or education, we can expect outcomes to be grossly unequal. Those born with severe health care or education needs would have to use unfair proportions of their resources, and it is still likely they would not have opportunity for equal outcomes.

The point is not that health care or education is morally more important. It is that the need for these is radically different. It now seems clearer to me than it did in 1981 that there may be ways of dealing with this gross difference in need in the health care arena. For example, if everyone had an entitlement to a health insurance plan with a premium of, say, $6,000 per family, and there were mandatory open enrollment and various controls for adverse selection, it might be less critical to treat health care as a unique benefit (Veatch 1997). I now see nothing unjust about letting people trade a portion of their $6,000 premium to buy a somewhat more slim coverage (provided the $6,000 would have bought coverage sufficient to give them opportunities for health equal insofar as possible to that of others). They could then use the savings in some other area that they prefer.[11] Giving an entitlement to enough coverage to have opportunities for well-being should be sufficient to preserve justice—or, at least, that is the direction in which I am moving.

5. Ranking, Balancing, and Specifying

The fifth and final area in which *Theory* needs to be revisited has to do with developments of how to resolve conflicts among principles. I remain convinced that my combination of ranking and balancing competing ethical principles is the only plausible strategy, the only one that squares with our considered moral judgments. Single-principle theories are terribly implausible, whether they are utilitarian, libertarian, or singly focused on the principle of justice. Even Pellegrino's single-principle theory focusing on patient beneficence, which tries to pack autonomy into its conceptualization, in my opinion, fails. Complete rank-ordering (lexical-ordering) is not plausible either. Balancing theories are fashionable. In one way or another, balancing is the recommended approach to conflict among principles in Beauchamp and Childress (2001, 18); Gert, Culver, and Clouser (1997, 57–58); and Brody (1988, 74–75).

   Balancing theories, however, have strange, sometimes offensive implications that seem not to square with our considered moral judgments. They would permit beneficence and nonmaleficence to overcome patient autonomy, leading to support of compulsory participation in dangerous medical research if only the expected benefits were great enough. They cannot explain why, in hundreds of cases in the United States, there has never been a single case in which competent patients were forced to undergo medical treatment against their wills. Autonomy at least takes absolute precedence over patient welfare. I am convinced it also takes precedence over social beneficence and nonmaleficence. While that seems implausible to many theorists, I believe that is because they fail to realize the leverage that comes from other principles. It is only when some other ethical principle that is not consequence-maximizing comes into play— some principle such as fidelity to promises, or avoiding killing, or justice— that autonomy can be overridden. This approach provides the caution of subordinating these duties related to respect for persons and justice to aggregate utility, while still providing a basis for overriding autonomy in exceptional cases.

Within the past decade the problem of conflict among principles has benefited from the addition of a theory of "specification" as a way of adding specificity to principles. Specification permits moving to more concrete domains of action, at which point one can generate rules for conduct that resolve conflict among principles, at least if one limits one's attention to the domain under consideration. I remain skeptical that specification really adds to the previously existing possibilities for generating rules based on generalizable features of classes of actions. The claim of the specificationists is that, if one limits attention to a specific domain, then specifications can be articulated that sort out the potential conflicts. The problem is that if, within a domain, one principle takes priority over another, one ought to be able to articulate the reason why that is so. And if that reason works in one domain, it is not clear why the same reason would not lead to the same priority in other domains as well, provided the facts are relevantly similar. The result, it would seem, is that reasons for resolving a conflict should not be restricted to a domain. The same reasons should lead to the same conclusions in relevantly similar situations, whether one is in one domain or another.[12]

CONCLUSION

When I began *A Theory of Medical Ethics*, we lived in a different world. There was nothing resembling a theoretical construction that could provide a systematic account of how to approach medical ethical problems. My approach, which rests on a recognition of the total inadequacy of the Hippocratic tradition, the development of a triple contract, a seven-principle theory including avoiding killing and justice, and a ranking combined with more limited balancing, is an approach to which I remain committed. The emergence of the alternative theoretical accounts put forward by many of the authors of the chapters in this volume presents new challenges to me. To that challenge I hope this essay provides an initial response.

NOTES

1. I have tried consistently to use the term *medicine* as synonymous with the field of health care, the way we use *education* to cover a broad sphere of social life, one that involves both professionals and lay people and many different roles within each of these two categories. Hence, I have always resisted ceding *medicine* to physicians or even to "health professionals." Medicine is, to me, the sphere of human life having to do with the well-being of the body. As such I have always held that most medical decisions are made by lay people—only some of whom

are in the patient or surrogate role. Most are made by lay people outside of any patient role, including those made by all of us about our own lives and the lives of people for whom we are responsible. Among the medical professions I include far more than "physicianing." I include nursing, pharmacy, dentistry, and the various allied health professions. From time to time I speak of physician ethics as a branch of medical ethics; and, among physician ethics, there is both profession-ally articulated physician ethics (such as that written by the AMA) and lay-articulated medical ethics (such as that written by judges, church groups, and individual scholars). I have described this use of the language in several places, including Veatch and Fry 1987.

2. From almost the beginning I had in mind someday doing case books in medical ethics for each of the health professions. Only recently have I completed that project (Veatch and Fry 1987; Rule and Veatch 1993; Veatch and Flack 1997; Veatch and Haddad 1999; Fry and Veatch 2000).

3. I reviewed the first edition for *The Hastings Center Report* in August of 1979 (Veatch 1979). From my habit of dating books when I start reading them, I know that I started reading the first edition on May 27, 1979, several months before submitting my manuscript to the publisher.

4. Carol Mason Spicer and I (Veatch and Mason 1987) defended this claim further by looking at the almost complete absence of interest in the Hippocratic oath in ancient Christianity and the clear understanding in the two instances of mention of the oath that Hippocratic ethics and Christian ethics were different.

5. Others have noted his influence not only in my metaethics, but also in my title.

6. I am more and more impressed with the postmodernist claim that there may be multiple, but noncontradictory, accounts of a reality.

7. Unless taking care of themselves were the only way to help their patients—a condition that not all self-improvement can meet.

8. One might claim that beneficence cannot justify such a killing because the killing would also violate the victim's autonomy. The claim would be that the combina-tion of the harm to the one killed plus the violation of his autonomy would outweigh the benefits for the rest of society. The problem with that more nuanced approach is that it still leaves one in a position where one ought to feel morally torn—between the good of the killing, on the one hand, and the harm combined with the autonomy violation on the other. We do not, however, feel morally torn by a proposal to kill a useless person in order to benefit society. We have a clear repulsion. Moreover, if good to society counts as even a prima facie defense of the killing, presumably there will eventually be a case in which someone is totally useless and the burden he creates is so great that the societal benefit of the killing can be said to override both the harm and the autonomy violation. If we add that the one to be killed is himself rather unhappy with life so that he himself says that, although he does not want to die, the loss would be only a modest harm, it seems it ought to be rather easy to justify the killing.

9. I am acutely aware of the dangers of claiming that the most vulnerable—the worst off—in society have special claims to have their interests served by killing them, but, with Paul Ramsey, I can imagine that someday there may be such a

case. Whether the risks of legalizing such killings are too great I leave for future public policy discussion.

10. This is true even though the food is consumed while the shelter is probably more stable, so that at some future time it will look like one person has more (a nice house) while the other has less. In fact, the other has the memories of better, more tasty foods and, assuming they start with equal resources, their opportunities for well-being should be considered equal.

11. There would still have to be practical limits, so that, for example, all persons would have access to emergency treatments if brought unconscious to an emergency room. The purpose is not to benefit that individual, but to serve the public good of making ER personnel wholeheartedly committed to patient care rather than requiring them to somehow determine whether the unconscious patient has insurance coverage for the care. Aside from these coverages that must be included to avoid untoward social effects and to avoid forcing people with known high risks into poor coverage plans, people can, I suggest, be permitted to choose among alternative coverages at alternative prices without treating them unjustly.

12. For example, although I reject Rawls's two principles of justice as an explication of what justice as a prima facie principle requires, it may work out that his principles are a very good approximation of what should happen when maximizing utility conflicts with justice interpreted in an egalitarian way. This suggests that, whenever justice conflicts with utility maximizing, a social practice should strive to promote opportunity for being as well off as possible, so that the only reason for tolerating unequal opportunities for welfare is that the worst off will be better off if there is inequality. It turns out not to be exactly the balancing of the competing principles that I end up supporting, but it is at least a plausible balancing. Rawls's two principles make much more sense as advice about how to balance justice and utility than as an interpretation of justice itself. Regardless of this claim that Rawls's principles are really a proposal to balance competing principles, it seems that he is correct that the formula is not domain specific. If he has good reasons for relating justice to utility in one domain, those same reasons would seem to apply for other domains in which the facts are similar.

References

American Medical Association. 2001. Principles of Medical Ethics (2001) of The American Medical Association.

Beauchamp, Tom L., and James F. Childress. 1979. *Principles of Biomedical Ethics.* 2d ed. New York: Oxford University Press.

———. 2001. *Principles of Biomedical Ethics.* 5th ed. New York: Oxford University Press.

Brody, Baruch. 1988. *Life and Death Decision Making.* New York: Oxford University Press.

Engelhardt, H. Tristram, Jr. 1986. *The Foundations of Bioethics.* New York: Oxford University Press.

———. 1996. *The Foundations of Bioethics.* 2d ed. New York: Oxford University Press.

Firth, Roderick. 1952. Ethical Absolutism and the Ideal Observer Theory. *Philosophy and Phenomenological Research* 12: 317–45.

Fry, Sara T., and Robert M. Veatch. 2000. *Case Studies in Nursing Ethics.* 2d ed. Sudbury, Mass.: Jones and Bartlett.

Gert, Bernard, Charles M. Culver, and K. Danner Clouser. 1997. *Bioethics: A Return to Fundamentals.* New York: Oxford University Press.

May, William F. 1975. Code, Covenant, Contract, or Philanthropy? *Hastings Center Report* 5: 29–38.

National Conference of Catholic Bishops. 2001. Ethical and Religious Directives for Catholic Health Care Services. Washington, D.C.: United States Catholic Conference.

Pellegrino, Edmund D., and David C. Thomasma. 1988. *For the Patient's Good: The Restoration of Beneficence in Health Care.* New York: Oxford University Press.

Ramsey, Paul. 1970. *The Patient as Person.* New Haven, Conn.: Yale University Press.

Rule, James T., and Robert M. Veatch. 1993. *Ethical Questions in Dentistry.* Chicago: Quintessence Books.

United States Catholic Conference, Department of Health Affairs. 1971. Ethical and Religious Directives for Catholic Health Facilities. Washington, D.C.: United States Catholic Conference.

Veatch, Robert M. 1976. *Death, Dying, and the Biological Revolution.* New Haven, Conn.: Yale University Press.

———. 1977. *Case Studies in Medical Ethics.* Cambridge, Mass.: Harvard University Press.

———. 1979. When Ethical Paths Converge. Review of *Principles of Biomedical Ethics* by Tom L. Beauchamp and James F. Childress. *Hastings Center Report* 9 (4): 48–49.

———. 1981. *A Theory of Medical Ethics.* New York: Basic Books.

———. 1994. Why Physicians Cannot Determine If Care Is Futile. *Journal of the American Geriatrics Society* 42 (8).

———. 1997. Single Payers and Multiple Lists: Must Everyone Get the Same Coverage in a Universal Health Plan? *Kennedy Institute of Ethics Journal* 7 (2): 153–69.

———. 2001. The Impossibility of a Morality Internal to Medicine. *Journal of Medicine and Philosophy* 26 (6): 621–42.

———. 2003. *The Basics of Bioethics.* 2d ed. Upper Saddle River, N.J.: Prentice-Hall, Inc.

Veatch, Robert M., and Harley E. Flack. 1997. *Case Studies in Allied Health Ethics.* Upper Saddle River, N.J.: Prentice Hall, Inc.

Veatch, Robert M., and Sara T. Fry. 1987. *Case Studies in Nursing Ethics.* Philadelphia: Lippincott.

Veatch, Robert M., and Amy Haddad. 1999. *Case Studies in Pharmacy Ethics.* New York: Oxford University Press.

Veatch, Robert M., and Carol G. Mason. 1987. Hippocratic vs. Judeo-Christian Medical Ethics: Principles in Conflict. *The Journal of Religious Ethics* 15: 86–105.

Veatch, Robert M., and Carol Mason Spicer. 1992. Medically Futile Care: The Role of the Physician in Setting Limits. *American Journal of Law & Medicine* 18, nos. 1, 2: 15–36.

———. 1993. Futile Care. *Health Progress* 74 (10): 22–27.

5

The Foundations of Bioethics: Rethinking the Meaning of Morality

H. TRISTRAM ENGELHARDT, JR.

ASSESSING THE ROOTS OF MORAL PLURALISM

In early 1966, I took a leave of absence from medical school to study philosophy. From a surgical clerkship at Charity Hospital in New Orleans I came to Klaus Hartmann's lectures on Immanuel Kant (Engelhardt 1994a). With me I brought philosophical puzzles, which were recast through explorations of Kant, Hegel, and Husserl. My medical-moral concerns were placed within foundational reflections on the nature of morality and metaphysics, as well as the development of eighteenth- and nineteenth-century thought. When I returned to complete my doctorate in medicine and begin research in the history of medicine, I found myself in 1971 in a concurrent academic position at Tulane, which included giving lectures on medical morality and the philosophy of medicine.[1] During this period, a news magazine report concerning the founding of the Kennedy Institute of Ethics came to my attention. A letter of inquiry, however, produced no response. This failure to engage the new Kennedy Institute's interest proved decisive. I continued to pursue issues in Continental philosophy (Engelhardt 1973a; Schutz and Luckmann 1973), as well as in the history and philosophy of medicine (Engelhardt 1975). My research had become more foundational than practical, just as the field of medical moral reflection was about to be baptized "bioethics."

This chapter places bioethics in terms of cultural developments that led to the emergence of secular, medical, moral reflections as a distinct field of intellectual investigation some thirty years ago. The contemporary phenomenon of bioethics, so I argue, should be understood as a late-modern intellectual undertaking about to go aground on the reefs of postmodernity. In this account, I give primary attention to *The*

Foundations of Bioethics, a volume begun in the mid-1970s and written twice (Engelhardt 1986, 1996). This volume is placed centrally because it developed as a critique of the dominant contemporary understanding of bioethics: the view that bioethics can uncontroversially build on a common morality or ethic, which can then be applied to or used within the context of medicine and the biomedical sciences. Where others saw an ethics for an applied ethics to apply or engage, I diagnosed controversy with no positive prognosis for resolution. *The Foundations of Bioethics* thus starts from what should be obvious: the controversies defining bioethics are the result of disputes engaged across moralities. The participants in the disputes meet as moral strangers, in the sense of sharing neither (1) sufficient basic premises and rules of moral inference, so as to resolve their controversies by sound rational argument, nor (2) a common understanding of who is in authority to resolve such controversies. *The Foundations of Bioethics* was undertaken as an attempt, despite this diversity, to secure something of the Enlightenment hope for a common morality able to bind persons as such.

The challenge proved formidable: the project of *The Foundations of Bioethics* confronted a paradoxical situation. On the one hand, bioethicists often claimed consensus in particular areas, yet the field was marked by substantive disagreements at the level of both theory and practice. This disarray was a matter of personal experience. When I set out over thirty years ago to make a presentation in bioethics, I had intended (being in those days a Roman Catholic) to frame a sound rational argument in opposition to abortion (Engelhardt 1971). To my dismay, it became clear that to secure the desired conclusions, initial, crucial, controversial, metaphysical, and moral premises needed first to be granted. This pox was not only on my house, but on all others as well. I came to accept what Hegel had recognized in the 1820s: morality is diverse and categorially multilevel (Engelhardt 1994b). The project of *The Foundations* was born.

It was in the face of the foundational moral controversies of the 1960s and 70s regarding rights, social justice, abortion, and various bioethics issues, along with a theoretical disarray as to how one might set them aside, that bioethics as an academic and practical field emerged. *The Foundations of Bioethics*, which raised fundamental questions about the possibility of a canonical, content-full, secular bioethics, took shape during the worldwide spread and acceptance of the new field of bioethics. The phenomenon of the field of bioethics having arrived nearly full-formed, and surely not in the condition of a newborn babe, can in part be explained by the profound hunger for what a profession of bioethics seemed to offer: concrete moral guidance. In the mid-1970s a moral vacuum had been created by the loss of taken-for-granted sources of moral community through (1) the deprofessionalization of medicine (Engelhardt 2001) and (2) the rapid secularization of American society. Into the 1960s, physicians had served as presumptive moral authorities regarding the proper conduct of their profession, claiming a moral wisdom and authority developed out of the experience of making life and death decisions with and about patients. When medicine came to be regarded as a trade rather than a socially recognized guild, it became less plausible to credit physicians' claims to an independent domain of moral insight and judgment, expressed in a professionally grounded medical ethics.[2] As a consequence, when the 1970s opened, the internal moral insights and claims of physicians seemed unjustifiable apart from their justification in general moral terms.

At the same time, America and the West, especially its cultural elites, were becoming post-Christian. America, which at the beginning of the twentieth century had been both *de facto* and *de jure* a Christian nation,[3] came through a number of court holdings and social upheavals in the 1950s and 60s to regard itself *de jure* as a secular polity.[4] This fundamental recasting of the character of the civil religion of America from that of a vague Protestant Christianity to that of a vague secular humanism disestablished the moral authority not only of priests and ministers, but also of rabbis and other religious authority figures. According to the emerging secular ethics, religious authorities qua religious authorities were no longer to opine in the public forum regarding the nature of medical morality (Rawls 1997). The public forum as secularized discouraged religious figures from advancing moral claims on the basis of their religious commitments (Hauerwas 1995). The now-dominant secular culture required them instead to translate their religious discourse into secular moral discourse. The secularization of the public forum fostered the moralization of public religious speech: religious concerns were translated into moral terms.

The secularization of medical morality gained strength in the wake of the post–Vatican II theological convulsions of Roman Catholicism. The Roman Catholic church had been the primary source of compendia on medical morality, having produced 300 years of manualist theological reflections, including, from the end of the nineteenth century, volumes in English addressing medical moral issues (Capellmann 1882; Coppens 1897). In the late 1960s, this moral research tradition collapsed (Kelly 1979). A centuries-old paradigm of theology, with its taken-for-granted epistemological assumptions, went into disarray. What had been an intact paradigm of medical moral reflection entered into crisis, bringing its examination of medical ethical issues into question.

The impact of secularization came with dramatic moral and metaphysical implications. Christianity revealed not only a human but also a cosmic history stretching from creation through the Fall to Redemption to the Second Coming and the final restoration of all things. A deep meaning for all history was disclosed. Things as creations of an omnipotent, personal, loving God have cosmic standing. After the death of God, events still happen in sequence, but that sequence is without an intrinsic meaning. With the loss of this experience of God, there is as well a loss of metaphysical orientation. The young Hegel[5] and Nietzsche understood this as "the greatest recent event—that 'God is dead', that belief in the Christian God has become unworthy of belief . . ." (Nietzsche 1960, 2:205, §343). In the face of the death of God and intractable moral diversity, nothing in the universe has enduring, independent meaning. Meaning, insofar as it exists, must instead be conveyed by persons within the interpersonal frameworks of particular narratives, discourses, or cultures. As Protagoras (c. 480–410 B.C.) observed, "Man is the measure of all things, of things that are that they are, and of things that are not that they are not" (Diogenes 1979, 2:463, 465). Persons are left in an apparently senseless universe with the task of making sense of the most important passages of human life. In this circumstance, humanist traditions fragment into numerous narratives of limited significance. As Gianni Vattimo has noted, "The death of God, which is at once the culmination and conclusion of metaphysics, is also the crisis of humanism" (Vattimo 1988, 8). Once God is dead for human culture, human nature loses canonical moral significance. Human nature and nature in general become objects for self-conscious reflection to address, objectify, and bring into question.

By the 1970s, as American society was confronting a powerful, effective, and costly complex of medical and biomedical technologies, the moral force of secularization had rendered quasi-theological orientation inaccessible. The culture had no canonical common vision to guide the development of its health care policy just as it needed to make very serious policy decisions. The society hungered after what it had lost, a guiding moral vision that could inform clinics, laboratories, and centers of health care policy. The Kennedy Institute of Ethics attempted to address this need. In its theoretical academic dimension, it nurtured scholars to articulate the moral vision that should guide health care and the biomedical sciences. In summers through "full immersion" courses and other venues, it trained practitioners who could apply this moral vision in hospitals and in governmental agencies. The result was a surrogate secular moral theology, along with secular priests in authority to give guidance (Engelhardt 2002). It was not simply that interests in medical-moral reflection were baptized under the rubric "bioethics." More fundamentally, bioethicists were ordained as in authority, at least in some narrow areas, to make moral determinations. Bioethicists as the practitioners of this new profession not only made themselves available (1) to analyze medical-moral concepts and claims, (2) to assess the soundness of the arguments involved, (3) to provide a geography of different moral approaches, and (4) to offer specific normative advice, now they were also (5) considered in limited ways in authority to pronounce on what should count as proper conduct (Wildes 1997; Kipnis 1997). The field and practice of bioethics came into existence to fill the moral and cultural vacuum that resulted from the deprofessionalization of medicine and the secularization of the West.

Georgetown and the Genesis

The first edition of *The Foundations* has roots in research begun at the Institute for Medical Humanities of the University of Texas Medical Branch in Galveston.[6] Even on that island I was influenced by associations with the Kennedy Institute. When interviewed for my position as Rosemary Kennedy Professor of the Philosophy of Medicine at Georgetown University (fall 1977 through December 1982), I made reference to a book I hoped soon to complete providing a systematic account of bioethics. My focus was still on redeeming some of the Enlightenment's hope for a generally justifiable, thick account of moral conduct. I only dimly acknowledged that this project would have to make reference to religious concerns with bioethical norms (Engelhardt 1973b). This latter task proved far more formidable than was at first apparent, leading me in the end on a spiritual journey from Rome to Antioch.

The inability in general secular terms to establish a particular morality as canonical became clearer over my five and a half years at the Kennedy Institute. During this time, James Childress and I were neighbors, often driving together to the Kennedy Institute, engaged in heated arguments concerning the appropriate content of a secular morality and bioethics. He was and is an affective friend, but surely a moral stranger. We sustained an extended dialogue, he a liberal cosmopolitan, and I a libertarian. With time it became obvious why he and Tom Beauchamp could employ middle-level principles to resolve controversies, while James Childress and I could use them only to see more clearly how deeply we disagreed. We were separated by different moral visions. I became convinced that, if one could identify anything worthy of the term principle, either as a chapter heading for matters moral or as a general source of moral content or structure, it could at best be very formal. Perhaps one could identify a right-making condition grounded in permission, and another grounded in the good, though in the end the good would always have to gain its content from a particular community, narrative, or moral perspective, or through particular agreements. Only later did I come to recognize the possibility of other substantively different dimensions of morality, such as that concerned with the holy. From these and other discussions at the Kennedy Institute, I turned to the task of laying out that sparse morality that can be shared by moral strangers.

The Foundations would need to account for unity, insofar as this was possible, as well as diversity in bioethics, which was manifest. As to the diversity, it was expressed in deep and ongoing controversies regarding the nature of appropriate conduct in matters such as third-party-assisted reproduction, abortion, the allocation of scarce resources, germline genetic engineering, cloning, organ sales, physician-assisted suicide, and euthanasia. Yet bioethics aspired to consensus. The field found itself directed to consensus not just because it had to resolve practical issues, but also because it was tied to political power. There was an implicit recognition that moral pronouncements could support particular health care policy agendas. Already in the mid-1970s, when I visited the Kennedy Institute as associate editor for the *Encyclopedia of Bioethics* (Reich 1978) as well as in the office of occasional lecturer (Engelhardt 1974), the emerging bond between political agendas and moral advocacy was salient. Due to the desire to derive public policy from bioethics, there was a vivid interest in proclaiming a consensus so as less problematically to justify that health care policy which was held to be acceptable by one's own faction. After all, bioethics is about politics and politics is about power.

This relationship between the content of a bioethics and particular political agendas is well illustrated by the various bioethics commissions. The attempt by the National Commission for the Protection of Human Subjects of Biomedical and Behavioral Research to frame a guiding bioethics illustrated that, if one selected individuals with similar ideological backgrounds, they could embrace common working moral premises and produce a consensus useful in anointing particular policy recommendations.[7] Thus, the subsequent President's Commission for the Study of Ethical Problems in Medicine and Biomedical and Behavioral Research of the Reagan years was careful not to endorse a right to health care

(President's Commission 1983). Also, as one would anticipate, Bill Clinton's National Bioethics Advisory Commission was replaced in late 2001 by President George W. Bush's Presidential Council on Bioethics. Each president has understood it to be in his interest to secure bioethicists to endorse, or at least not radically bring into question, his view of morally appropriate biomedical conduct and health care policy. Had commissions compassed in their membership something of the full spectrum of moral visions, ranging from socialists to libertarians, impassioned atheists to fundamentalist Christians, the result would have been a special genre of philosophical seminar, not a forum for the endorsement of particular policies. In short, there are ideological reasons to avoid real diversity and to create the appearance of consensus. If one acknowledges the breadth and depth of controversy, then bioethics is defined by moral diversity.

BIOETHICS AND THE MORAL EPISTEMOLOGICAL CRISIS OF POSTMODERNITY

The difference that separates moralities defines postmodernity's challenge to traditional views of morality: two cardinal characteristics of that challenge have been the focus of both editions of *The Foundations of Bioethics*. They are at the core of the difficulties at the roots of contemporary moral theory and bioethics. They are the source of the battles in the culture wars. The first is the manifest plurality of moralities. There is a plurality of moralities in the very strong sense of incompatible sets of considered settled judgments and evaluational frameworks sustaining competing understandings of what should count as appropriate action. A family of concerns about appropriate conduct may be identifiable, so that one can talk of the human moral project. Still, *de facto* one is confronted with a plurality of moralities advancing conflicting and incompatible claims— for example, claims about the appropriateness or inappropriateness of abortion, the adoption of a one-tier health care system as in Canada, and the propriety of germline genetic engineering. Such disagreements among moralities are substantive. They involve conflicts among different views as to when it is appropriate or inappropriate to kill human life and/or coercively restrict the free purchase of health services.

As *The Foundations* took shape, the importance of distinguishing between a common morality and common elements among different moralities became clear.[8] A common human morality (as opposed to a canonical morality that is the standard for human conduct, albeit not generally recognized), were it to exist, would be a shared understanding regarding appropriate conduct. Analyses of different moralities may identify moral concerns shared by all humans due to the common human context and the character of embodiment, such as that humans *inter alia* are concerned about pain, pleasure, property, and death. However, different moralities support different views as to when pains and pleasures of particular sorts are appropriate, as well as regarding the circumstances under which it is good to take human life or property. It may be the case that across moralities, all else being equal (i.e., in the absence of any consideration in its favor), it is held wrong to lie, kill, break promises, or coercively take the property of others. What distinguishes moralities are the settled judgments they support regarding the general conditions under which killing, the taking of property, the telling of falsehoods, etc., are appropriate or inappropriate. Only within a particular morality is one instructed regarding the general classes of circumstances in which it is in fact obligatory or forbidden to kill humans, lie, or take their property. A morality specifies when it is appropriate to act in particular ways about particular focal concerns of human life (e.g., pain, pleasure, sexuality, trust, property, and killing). Such foci of "moral concern," if not ordered and interpreted in a common normative framework, constitute only points for moral controversy. They are not elements of a common morality, as disputes regarding the moral propriety of abortion, capital punishment, dueling, and euthanasia illustrate. Common norms of moral concern do not a common morality make. Common moral elements identify only moral concerns out of which different moralities are structured. It therefore became clear that to speak of humans sharing a common morality is not only unfounded but also strategically deceptive. It obscures the depth and importance of human moral disagreement, which may in particular circumstances be an ideological device for rallying political support for one public policy option and against other, competing options.

Differences among moralities are even starker if some recognize that moral decisions have eternal significance. When the field of moral dispute compasses moralities for which proper conduct leads to union with a fully transcendent God, the participants in the controversies can be separated by deeply conflicting views of the significance of morality itself. The matter is complicated by the circumstance that in some religious moral accounts there is no practice of moral philosophy parallel to and corrective upon the accepted account of right conduct. Right conduct is understood as a spiritual therapy, not as an end in itself (Hierotheos 1994). Because of their focus on a transcendent personal deity and norms experienced in revelation, neither Orthodox Judaism nor Orthodox Christianity possesses a moral theology or bioethics in the sense that emerged in the secular or the Christian West: a discursive rational reflection on right conduct with an internal dynamic of its own.[9] Since the interpretive framework or metaphysical background of a morality conveys meaning to a morality (e.g., that living a good but not holy life is insufficient for salvation), moralities may be distinguished not just in terms of their articulation of particular immanent moral concerns or "norms," but in terms of the meaning that background metaphysical frameworks give to such concerns or "norms."

Elizabeth Anscombe recognized the metaphysical roots of moral differ-ence and the cleft it grounds between traditional theistic moral under-standings and contemporary morality. Different metaphysical assumptions define different competing moralities. If traditional Christian morality is taken as the standard, then contemporary non-theistic morality is only incompletely a morality.

> It is as if the notion "criminal" were to remain when criminal law and criminal courts had been abolished and forgotten. A Hume discovering this situation might conclude that there was a special sentiment, expressed by "criminal," which alone gave the word its sense. (Anscombe 1958, 6)

In its account of moral pluralism, *The Foundations of Bioethics* acknowl-edges moral diversity without embracing a metaphysical skepticism regard-ing the existence of moral truth. Instead, there are grounds for a moral epistemological skepticism about the capacities of secular moral rationality to know when one knows moral truth.

This skepticism is grounded in the second characteristic of the contem-porary moral condition: the limits of secular moral epistemology. There is a growing recognition of the impossibility of securing intellectual foun-dations that can deliver a canonical warrant for one particular morality vis-à-vis all competing others without begging the question, arguing in a circle, or engaging in infinite regress. Without begging the question one cannot deliver a particular foundation for a particular morality. To justify a particular ordering of moral principles or core moral values, one must already have in the background a particular evaluative vision to justify the appropriate ordering. One cannot know when one knows the correct morality without begging the question of the nature of moral knowledge.

This state of affairs can be illustrated by examining different approaches to justifying a particular moral vision. For instance, given the appropriate ranking of such cardinal values as liberty, equality, prosperity, and security, one will embrace something like the social democratic vision of John Rawls (Rawls 1971, 1993) or instead a soft dictatorial capitalism, a la Singapore (Fan 1997; Alora and Lumitao 2001). Without already having a canonical perspective, one cannot in a principled fashion determine which moral sense or moral intuitions should guide. After all, normatively to specify the content of morality, one must know how to rank consequences, how to compare the satisfaction of rational versus impassioned preferences, how to decide among different discount rates for preference satisfaction over time, as well as how to select the correct moral sense or moral rationality to guide hypothetical choosers, contractors, or rational moral choosers, etc. One cannot by sound rational argument deliver a secular surrogate for the rational and universalist morality of Western Christianity without the equivalent of a secular revelation (i.e., concession) of initial moral commitments. The West has been returned to the ancient world and its obvious polytheism of moral diversity. The contentions in favor of a universal content-full morality grounded in sound rational argument have failed.

My reflections regarding moral controversy, the difficulty of consensus, and the circumstances under which moral controversies can be resolved by sound rational argument acquired further substance through a series of rich, and for me influential, meetings, which included Alasdair Mac-Intyre and later Tom Beauchamp. These discussions were held at the Hastings Center from 1975 through 1982. They produced a series of volumes examining the issue of and the character of scientific controversies marked by a heavy moral and political overlay (Callahan and Engelhardt 1981; Engelhardt and Callahan 1976, 1977, 1978, 1980), under the general rubric of "The Foundations of Ethics and Its Relationship to Science." Further discussions culminated in a volume that appeared one year after the first edition of *The Foundations of Bioethics* (Engelhardt and Caplan 1987). This collection of studies again showed that moral diversity is substantive and not able to be set aside by sound rational argument. Secular moral reflection was not able to deliver a surrogate for the canonical moral revelation that had once been presumed at the foundations of Christendom. To ask for a common moral vision justifiable in general secular terms turned out to be a secular restatement of a Christian hope in matters theological, now stated in a secular context where such hope was unjustifiable. The secular displacement of a theological concern produced a project that was insoluble: the secular, rational justification of a particular canonical, content-full morality.

BIOETHICS IN THE RUINS OF WESTERN CHRISTENDOM: SECULAR PRIESTS AND THE HUNGER FOR MORAL GUIDANCE

Faced with an irresolvable plurality of moral visions, the secular moral choice of any particular account is contingent. Here *The Foundations of Bioethics* agrees with Richard Rorty regarding both the content of particular secular moralities, as well as the morality that is to bind moral strangers. "We can keep the notion of 'morality' just insofar as we can cease to think of morality as the voice of the divine part of ourselves . . ." (Rorty 1989, 59). Even human dignity, which is etymologically tied to a bestowed honorific status, such as that bestowed by God at creation (Genesis 1:26), loses its depth as morality becomes understood in fully secular terms. The announcement of content-full human rights is bereft of any divine tone. Morality becomes a human expedient articulated in diverse and competing forms.

The Foundations of Bioethics recognizes the force of secularization and the consequent loss of an ultimate orientation as being more significant than Rorty admits. *The Foundations* denies the view that, despite this rupture, we can nevertheless continue to think of "the voice of ourselves as members of a [secular moral] community, speakers of a common [secular moral] language" (Rorty 1989, 59), providing a canonical guide for moral choice. The objectifying power of self-reflective consciousness brings into question every particular community with its particular morality. Any particular ranking of right-making principles or core values could always have been otherwise. No particular, secular moral narrative can be generally normative. It is always one among many possible competing moral narratives: a polytheism of moral perspectives dominates. Here, Vattimo understands the challenge much more clearly and fully than does Rorty: "Atheism appears in this light as another catastrophic Tower of Babel . . ." (Vattimo 1988, 31). Postmodernity is that Babel. Atheism is the herald of the end of modernity. It is for this reason that even the French Republic born of the Revolution preserved a place for deism. Thus, too, Kant acknowledged the cardinal role of God as the guarantor of a unique moral perspective. Monotheism secures the plausibility of a privileged moral perspective over against a polytheism of moralities. Kant appreciated that, in the absence of God, the unity of motivation and justification for moral action is broken (Immanuel Kant, *Critique of Pure Reason*, A813 = B841). The good and the right can be at odds, so that doing the right can, on balance, harm. Without the metaphysical anchor of God, the genesis, justification, and motivation of morality are sundered. Kant therefore introduced his as-if postulates of God and immortality. At the end of the Enlightenment and on the threshold of postmodernity, Kant attempted to secure an at least as-if metaphysical unity for the moral life (Kant 1902, vol. 5, 125).

The first and second editions of *The Foundations of Bioethics*, as well as *Bioethics and Secular Humanism* (Engelhardt 1991), only incompletely appreciated these developments. *The Foundations* did provide a critique of the drive to establish a secular moral orthodoxy as a surrogate for the religious faith now lost. It showed why a secular orthodoxy cannot succeed in establishing a content-full, canonical, moral account. As a positive project, *The Foundations* justified a framework for morally authoritative collaboration among moral strangers. It was able as well to reconstruct the moral grounding of, and therefore establish the moral authority for, those practices that through permission can bind moral strangers, as by contracts, the market, and limited democracy. A more substantive account of the genesis of our contemporary postmodern predicament as well as of the possibilities for a content-full morality had to await *The Foundations of Christian Bioethics* (Engelhardt 2000).

It was fourteen years after the publication of the first edition of *The Foundations of Bioethics* that the exploration of the theological roots of moral diversity gave issue to *The Foundations of Christian Bioethics*. However, a first step in its direction had already been taken in the 1970s and early 1980s as I engaged James Childress and Richard McCormick, S.J., in reflections regarding the possibility of a Christian bioethics. At the Kennedy Institute, I had been introduced to Francesc Abel, S.J., who was at that time exploring issues of Roman Catholic bioethics for the International Study Group in Bioethics of the International Federation of Catholic Universities (Abel 2001). Abel asked if I would be interested in participating. At that time I said no. However, in the mid-1980s a second invitation came from John Collins Harvey, to whom I will remain eternally grateful. First unofficially and then officially, from 1987 to 1991 I served as a member of the steering committee for this study group. This choice was philosophically and theologically decisive: it engaged me in some seven years of reflection concerning the foundational assumptions of Western philosophy and theology, the result of which brought me to the Orthodox Christian catechumenate in Great Lent of 1991.

Four times over, this latter book is intimately tied to *The Foundations of Bioethics*. First, *The Foundations of Christian Bioethics* illustrates the possibility of a community of moral friends, in contrast to the procedural morality of moral strangers. Indeed, from the perspective of that volume, it provides *the* canonical exemplar, in comparison with which all others are deficient examples. Second, it locates more fully than *The Foundations of Bioethics* the extent to which Western Christian moral understandings lie at the root not only of Western European modernity and the Enlightenment's philosophical aspirations, but of the crisis of postmodernity as well. Third, it discloses radical moral difference. To paraphrase Patriarch Bartholomew I of New Rome in his presentation "Joyful Light"[10] at Georgetown University (October 21, 1997), *The Foundations of Christian Bioethics* supplies an account of "the manner in which [both Western culture and Western Christianity have become] ontologically different" from the Christianity of the first seven Ecumenical Councils (Bartholomew 1997, 2). A morality grounded in the noetic experience of union with ultimate Truth does not support a bioethics in the sense of a canon of appropriate conduct in health care justifiable in discursive moral-philosophical terms. In the first sense, morality is about relationship with God and through God with other persons. In the second sense, morality is an impersonal quasi-juridical standard for appropriate conduct. The second edition of *The Foundations* (Engelhardt 1996) underscored that the morality of moral strangers reflects the default position for moral discourse in the absence of grace and in the face of a plurality of moral rationalities.

A CONTENTIOUS CONCLUSION: THREE VARIETIES OF MORALITY AND THEIR BIOETHICS

The Foundations of Bioethics and its companion volume *The Foundations of Christian Bioethics* offer three quite different appreciations of morality and its foundations. Each presupposes for its grounding what can be termed, to use antique terminology, a different human faculty. The first, Western Christian and most secular philosophical reflection, presupposes discursive rationality as key. The second, my thin proposal in *The Foundations of Bioethics*, places the will centrally as grounding the morality of moral strangers. Finally, the Christianity of the first millennium understands the cardinal faculty to be the *nous*, a faculty largely unaddressed and thoroughly misunderstood in most Western theology. It is this understanding of morality that is sketched by *The Foundations of Christian Bioethics*.

The first has its roots in second-millennium Western Christian and Western philosophical aspirations via rational reflection to disclose either directly or indirectly the canons of appropriate conduct. Western Christianity was born of this second-millennium marriage of faith and reason.[11]

Western Christian and secular natural-law approaches to morality held out hope that discursive reason could disclose the canons for proper conduct. Even when reason was not considered the source of moral content, it was regarded as the appropriate arbiter of rational discourse. The avenue has become a cul-de-sac. *Pace* such theorists as Jürgen Habermas and his discourse ethics (Habermas 1981), all turns out only to be an issue of where one begs the question with respect to a particular moral rationality that must be granted either in the initial premises or in one's account of the character of the rationality of rational discourse. Sound rational moral arguments depend on first embracing a particular notion of moral rationality. Of course, that is what is at issue: understandings of moral rationality are plural.

The second source for a foundation for bioethics is the will: the will to act together with moral authority drawn from the concurrence of collaborators. Will as permission is the source of the authority that binds individuals in contracts, the free market, and limited democracies. This sparse morality for moral strangers presumes no common understanding of substantive morality. Indeed, it must eschew content (e.g., a particular ordering of moral values and principles) so as to bind moral strangers. This sparse morality provides a transcendental condition in the sense of a necessary condition for the possibility of moral strangers collaborating with common moral authority. As such, this morality offers only a procedural grammar for moral discourse among moral strangers. It does not provide motivation, much less justification, for entering into this discourse. Many may, and do, out of a multitude of diverse motivations, and in terms of different moral views, enter into contracts, trade in the market, and sustain limited democracies. However, one cannot in general secular moral terms show why it would be wrong or bad if they refused. All one can do is indicate a grammar for discourse among moral strangers (i.e., persons who do not share a common, content-full morality), should they wish to enter with an authority shared by all who consent to participate. This discourse generates spontaneous orders that emerge out of webs of content-rich agreements that generate particular peaceable agreements to collaborate.

Finally, with reference to *The Foundations of Christian Bioethics*, Patriarch Bartholomew offers an invitation to enter into a quite different understanding of morality: the one that lies at the basis of this last volume. He points to the life of first-millennium Christianity, living still. At its core lies a canonical, noetic experience "confirmed by grace in the heart [Heb. 13:9]" (Bartholomew 1997, 3). Those who are willing to recognize the cosmos as the creation of a personal, omniscient, omnipotent God can, through right worship, come to discern in that creation not merely the signs of God but the presence of God. Out of an experience of that God, they can orient themselves in a rightly structured moral understanding (Sophrony 1988), a canonical, content-full morality. This is not the place to say more about this noetic grounding of morality, only to indicate its presence like a door to be opened, through repentance and the response of a personal God. This grounding of substantive morality within rightly oriented worship leading through purification to illumination and union with God discloses a morality quite different from what can be offered either by discursive rationality or free choice. *The Foundations of Bioethics* and *The Foundations of Christian Bioethics* have sought to take moral diversity and the limits of secular moral rationality seriously and to indicate the consequences for both secular moral reflection and Christian theology.

NOTES

1. During medical school (1963–65, 1970–72), my encounters with medical ethics were restricted to lectures by wise physicians, clerics, and one presentation by Joseph Fletcher at Touro Infirmary in New Orleans. With the arrogance of the young, I explained to Fletcher that he had misconstrued Kant. He responded that he was interested in recasting the contemporary moral context, not framing precious, erudite distinctions.

2. During the twentieth century, medicine was transformed from a *de facto* guild to a trade through the force of Supreme Court holdings. See, for example, *American Medical Association v. United States*, 317 U.S. 519 (1943), and *American Medical Association v. Federal Trade Commission*, 638 F. 2d 443 (2d Cir. 1980).

3. Until the mid-twentieth century, the Supreme Court characterized Americans as a Christian people. *United States v. Macintosh*, 283 U.S. 605 (1931).

4. In the 1950s, the Supreme Court begins to step away from characterizing America as a Christian polity. *Everson v. Board of Education*, 330 U.S. 1 (1947); *Tessim Zorach v. Andrew G. Clauson et al.*, 343 U.S. 306, 96 L ed 954, 72 Sup. Ct. 679 (1951).

5. As a diagnosis of European culture, Hegel in *Glauben und Wissen* (1802) announced that "God Himself is dead" (Hegel 1977, 190). In 1795, Hegel had recognized this cultural rupture in *Das Leben Jesu*, which recasts Christ into a philosopher who *inter alia* opines, "Only this voice from heaven can instruct you concerning the higher demands of reason. . . . Reason does not condemn the natural impulses, but governs and refines them" (Hegel 1984, 108).

6. My turn to bioethics was encouraged by an invitation from the National Commission for the Protection of Human Subjects of Biomedical and Behavioral Research to provide a background paper regarding the foundations of bioethics. I offered

three basic ethical principles. "A. One should respect human subjects as free agents out of a duty to such subjects to acknowledge their right to respect as free agents. B. One should foster the best interests of individual human subjects. C. One should have concern to maximize the benefits accruable to society from research involving human subjects, taking into particular regard interest in values such as (1) the amelioration of the human condition through advances in the biomedical and behavioral sciences and technologies; (2) preservation of human autonomy as a general value; (3) increase in knowledge apart from any consideration of its application to the amelioration of the human condition; (4) the personal satisfaction of human subjects derived from their feeling of having contributed to the common good or to the advancement of human knowledge by participation in research" (Engelhardt 1978, pp. 8-5, 8-6).

7. Despite the National Commission's "consensus," the subject of its first report remains a focus of sustained public controversy (National Commission 1975).

8. "Morality" is used to identify a framework of considered, settled moral understandings that provide guidance as to what behavior will be held blameworthy or praiseworthy, good or bad, virtuous or vicious.

9. The independent authority of philosophical reflection in reshaping theology is a feature marking the emergence of Western Christianity. Thus, John Paul II defines moral theology as "a science which accepts and examines Divine Revelation while at the same time responding to the demands of human reason" (John Paul II 1993, § 29, p. 47). Consider, also: "Through the course of centuries, theology has progressively developed into a true and proper science. The theologian must therefore be attentive to the epistemological requirements of his discipline, to the demands of rigorous critical standards and thus to a rational verification of each stage of his research" (Congregation for the Doctrine of the Faith 1990).

10. The Ecumenical Patriarch's address carries the title of the vesperal hymn sung (or recited) as the priest completes the little entrance through the Royal Doors, beginning a new liturgical day.

11. First-millennium Christianity's view of the role of philosophy and theology is Pauline. "For it hath been written: 'I will destroy the wisdom of the wise, and will set at nought the comprehension of the intelligent.' . . . Did not God make foolish the wisdom of this world? . . . [I]n the wisdom of God, the world knew not God through its wisdom . . ." (I Cor. 1:19–21). Drawing on this Pauline view, St. John Chrysostom argues that discursive theological reflection leads away from right worship and right belief to heresy. "Let heretics hearken to the voice of the Spirit, for such is the nature of reasonings. . . . For being ashamed to allow of faith, and to seem ignorant of heavenly things, they involve themselves in the dust-cloud of countless reasonings" (Chrysostom 1994, vol. 11, pp. 349–50). In contrast, John Paul II underscores: "I wish to repeat clearly that the study of philosophy is fundamental and indispensable to the structure of theological studies and to the formation of candidates for the priesthood" (John Paul II 1998, §62, p. 93). Western Christianity regards theology as a discursive or merely contemplative endeavor. "The chief purpose of theology is to *provide an understanding of Revelation and the content of faith.* The very heart of theological enquiry will thus be the contemplation of the mystery of the Triune God" (John

Paul II 1998, §93, p. 136). In contrast, Metropolitan Hierotheos of Nafpaktos argues, "The philosophers philosophized by conjecture, imagination, and having reason at the centre, while for the holy Fathers the nous was the centre. They first purified their hearts of passions, and their nous was illuminated. . . . Theology is not related to philosophy, but more akin to medicine. And indeed we observe that all the heretics through the ages used philosophy, whereas the holy Fathers lived hesychasm" (Hierotheos 1998, 34). In this light, John Paul II's interpretation of St. Paul's reflections regarding the "eyes of the mind" and their relationship to reason must be seen within the theological paradigms of the second millennium (John Paul II 1998, § 22, p. 34).

REFERENCES

Abel, Francesc. 2001. *Bioética: Orígenes, presente y futuro*. Madrid: Fundacíon Mapfre Medicina.

Alora, Angeles Tan, and Josephine Lumitao, eds. 2001. *Beyond a Western Bioethics: Voices from the Developing World*. Washington, D.C.: Georgetown University Press.

Anscombe, G. E. M. 1958. Modern Moral Philosophy. *Philosophy* 33: 1–19.

Bartholomew I, Ecumenical Patriarch. 1997. Joyful Light. Address delivered at Georgetown University, October 21.

Callahan, Daniel, and H. T. Engelhardt, Jr., eds. 1981. *The Roots of Ethics*. New York: Plenum Press.

Capellmann, Carl. 1882. *Pastoral Medicine*, translated by William Dassel. New York: F. Pustet, orig. 1877.

Chrysostom, St. John. 1994. Homily II on Romans I.8, II.17. *Nicene and Post-Nicene Fathers*, First Series, edited by Philip Schaff. Peabody, Mass.: Hendrickson Publishers. Vol. 11.

Congregation for the Doctrine of the Faith. 1990. Instruction on the Ecclesial Vocation of the Theologian. *Origins* 20: 120.

Coppens, Charles. 1897. *Moral Principles and Medical Practice*. 3d ed. New York: Benziger Brothers.

Diogenes Laertius. 1979. *Protagoras* IX, 51. *Lives of Eminent Philosophers*, translated by R. D. Hicks. Cambridge, Mass.: Harvard University Press.

Engelhardt, Jr., H. T. 1971. Abortion: Some Philosophical Reflections. Lecture given at State University of New York, Stony Brook, November 15.

———. 1973a. *Mind-Body: A Categorial Relation*. The Hague: Martinus Nijhoff.

———. 1973b. Reflections on Religion and Medicine. *University Medical* [University of Texas Medical Branch] (Christmas): 15–16.

———. 1974. Medicine and the Concept of Person. The Expanding Universe of Modern Medicine, Matchette Foundation Lecture Series, Georgetown University, Washington, D.C., November 18.

———. 1975. John Hughlings Jackson and the Mind-Body Relation. *Bulletin of the History of Medicine*, 49: 137–51.

————. 1978. Basic Ethical Principles in the Conduct of Biomedical and Behavioral Research Involving Human Subjects. *The Belmont Report*, Appendix Vol. 1, Department of Health, Education, and Welfare, Publ. No. (12) 78-0013, section 8, pp. 1–45.

————. 1986. *The Foundations of Bioethics*. New York: Oxford University Press.

————. 1991. *Bioethics and Secular Humanism*. Philadelphia: Trinity Press International.

————. 1994a. Klaus Hartmann and G. W. F. Hegel: A Personal Postscript. In *Hegel Reconsidered*, edited by H. T. Engelhardt, Jr., and Terry Pinkard. Dordrecht: Kluwer.

————. 1994b. Sittlichkeit and Postmodernity: An Hegelian Reconstruction of the State. In *Hegel Reconsidered*, edited by H. T. Engelhardt, Jr., and Terry Pinkard. Dordrecht: Kluwer.

————. 1996. *The Foundations of Bioethics*. 2d ed. New York: Oxford University Press.

————. 2000. *The Foundations of Christian Bioethics*. Lisse, Netherlands: Swets & Zeitlinger.

————. 2001. The Deprofessionalization of Medicine in the United States: From Guild to Managed Care. *Occasional Paper Series No. 9*, City University of Hong Kong (August): 1–13.

————. 2002. The Ordination of Bioethicists as Secular Moral Experts. *Social Philosophy & Policy* 19(2): 59–82.

Engelhardt, Jr., H. T., and Daniel Callahan, eds. 1976. *Science, Ethics, and Medicine*. Hastings-on-Hudson, N.Y.: Hastings Center.

————. 1977. *Knowledge, Value, and Belief*. Hastings-on-Hudson, N.Y.: Hastings Center.

————. 1978. *Morals, Science, and Sociality*. Hastings-on-Hudson, N.Y.: Hastings Center.

————. 1980. *Knowing and Valuing*. Hastings-on-Hudson, N.Y.: Hastings Center.

Engelhardt, Jr., H. T., and Arthur Caplan, eds. 1987. *Scientific Controversies: A Study in the Resolution and Closure of Disputes Concerning Science and Technology*. New York: Cambridge University Press.

Fan, Ruiping. 1997. Three Levels of Problems in Cross-Cultural Explorations of Bioethics. In *Japanese and Western Bioethics*, edited by Kazumasa Hoshino. Dordrecht: Kluwer.

Habermas, Jürgen. 1981. *Theorie des kommunikativen Handelns*. Frankfurt: Suhrkamp. 2 vols.

Hauerwas, Stanley. 1995. How Christian Ethics Became Medical Ethics: The Case of Paul Ramsey. *Christian Bioethics* 1: 11–28.

Hegel, G. W. F. 1977. *Faith and Knowledge*, translated by Walter Cerf. Albany: State University of New York Press.

———. 1984. *Three Essays, 1793–1795*, translated by Peter Fuss and John Dobbins. Notre Dame, Ind.: University of Notre Dame Press.

Hierotheos of Nafpaktos. 1994. *Orthodox Psychotherapy*, translated by Esther Williams. Levadia, Greece: Birth of the Theotokos Monastery.

———. 1998. *The Person in the Orthodox Tradition*, translated by Esther Williams. Levadia, Greece: Birth of the Theotokos Monastery.

John Paul II. 1993. *Veritatis Splendor*. Vatican City: Libreria Editrice Vaticana.

———. 1998. *Fides et Ratio*. Vatican City: Libreria Editrice Vaticana.

Kant, Immanuel. 1902. *Kants Werke*. Berlin: Preussische Akademie der Wissenschaften.

Kelly, David F. 1979. *The Emergence of Roman Catholic Medical Ethics in North America*. New York: Edwin Mellen Press.

Kipnis, Kenneth. 1997. Confessions of an Expert Ethics Witness. *Journal of Medicine and Philosophy* 22: 325–43.

National Commission for the Protection of Human Subjects of Biomedical and Behavioral Research. 1975. *Research on the Fetus*. Publ. no. (OS) 76-127, 128. Washington, D.C.: Department of Health, Education, and Welfare.

Nietzsche, Friedrich. 1960. *Die fröhliche Wissenschaft*. Munich: Carl Hanser Verlag.

President's Commission for the Study of Ethical Problems in Medicine and Biomedical and Behavioral Research. 1983. *Securing Access to Health Care*. Washington, D.C.: U.S. Government Printing Office.

Rawls, John. 1971. *A Theory of Justice*. Cambridge, Mass.: Harvard University Press.

———. 1993. *Political Liberalism*. New York: Columbia University Press.

———. 1997. The Idea of Public Reason Revisited. *University of Chicago Law Review* 64: 765–807.

Reich, Warren, ed. 1978. *Encyclopedia of Bioethics*. New York: Macmillan Free Press.

Rorty, Richard. 1989. *Contingency, Irony, and Solidarity*. New York: Cambridge University Press.

Schutz, Alfred, and Thomas Luckmann. 1973. *The Structures of the Life-World*, translated by Richard M. Zaner and H. T. Engelhardt, Jr. Evanston, Ill.: Northwestern University Press.

Sophrony, Archimandrite. 1988. *We Shall See Him as He Is*. Essex: Monastery of St. John the Baptist.

Vattimo, Gianni. 1988. *The End of Modernity*, translated by Jon R. Snyder. Baltimore, Md.: Johns Hopkins University Press.

Wildes, Kevin Wm. 1997. Healthy Skepticism: The Emperor Has Very Few Clothes. *Journal of Medicine and Philosophy* 22: 365–71.

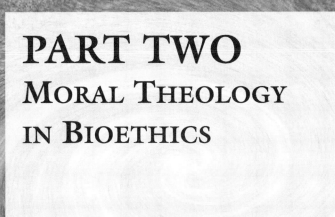

PART TWO
MORAL THEOLOGY
IN BIOETHICS

The Catholic Moral Tradition
in Bioethics

CHARLES E. CURRAN

As a Roman Catholic moral theologian I work out of a tradition that understands itself to be a *living* tradition that changes and develops. This essay will proceed in three stages—the prehistory of bioethics with special attention to medical ethics in the Roman Catholic perspective; my approach to bioethics in the early 1970s; and a reflection looking back on what has developed in Catholic bioethics since that time and looking forward to what might transpire in the future.

André Hellegers, the esteemed founder of the Kennedy Institute in 1971 and a good friend, invited me to spend the 1972 calendar year as a senior research scholar at the Institute. That year I wrote a monograph—*Politics, Medicine, and Christian Ethics: A Dialogue with Paul Ramsey* (1973). My colleagues that year at the Kennedy Institute, in addition to André Hellegers, the founder, and LeRoy Walters, the director of the Institute, were Francesc Abel, John Connery, Richard McCormick, Gene Outka, and Warren Reich. These were all scholars with a background in Christian ethics, and five of the seven come out of the tradition of Catholic moral theology. Many might expect a predominance of Catholic scholars in a Catholic university in 1972, but the fact that Georgetown is a Catholic university does not adequately explain the strong Catholic presence and interest in medical ethics in 1972.

PREHISTORY OF BIOETHICS

By 1960, medical ethics was a well-developed subdiscipline of moral theology in the Roman Catholic tradition. Books on medical ethics existed in the major European languages (Bonnar 1939; Healy 1956; Kelly 1958; Kenny 1952; Niedermeyer 1935; O'Donnell 1956; Paquin 1957; Payen 1935; Pujiula 1953; Scremin 1953). Periodicals devoted to medical ethics existed in many of the same languages—*Arzt und Christ, Cahiers Laënnec, Catholic Medical Quarterly, Linacre Quarterly*, and *Saint-Luc médicale*. Catholic medical ethics was strong in the United States especially due to the courses on medical ethics in Catholic medical and nursing schools and the textbooks used for these courses. With the exception of a very few Protestants, neither religious ethicists nor philosophical ethicists were interested in medical ethics at this time.

This historical situation raises three questions: (1) Why were Roman Catholic scholars interested in medical ethics? (2) Why were other ethicists not interested in medical ethics? (3) What explains the great interest in medical ethics and the tremendous growth of bioethics since?

WHY WERE ROMAN CATHOLICS SO INTERESTED IN MEDICAL ETHICS BEFORE 1960?

Historically, Roman Catholicism has insisted on the need to respond to the gift of God's love with a change of heart and to show such a change in good actions in daily life. The Catholic tradition has insisted on both faith and works. The Catholic emphasis on works at times went too far, even to the point of Pelagianism—the heresy that human beings save themselves by their own works and are not saved by God's gift. The sacrament of penance in the Catholic tradition underscored the importance of works. From the time of the Fourth Lateran Council in 1215, Catholics were obliged to confess their mortal sins at least once a year (Denzinger et al. 1963). Appropriate books came into existence to describe the good actions required in life and to point out the wrong or sinful actions. The most famous of these texts in the fifteenth century was the *Summa* of St. Antoninus, the Archbishop of Florence (1389–1459). In the third volume of a huge four-volume work, Antoninus considers the duties and obligations of people according to their different states in life— married people, virgins and widows, temporal rulers, soldiers, lawyers, doctors, merchants, judges, craftworkers, and many others. The duties and obligations of physicians include the following: competence, diligence, care for the patient, the obligation to tell the dying patient of his or her condition, the proper fee or salary for the doctor, the duty to care for the sick even when they cannot pay, and the obligation not to proscribe things against the moral law such as fornication and abortion (Florentini 1740, 277–92).

One illustration will show the very realistic practical wisdom of Antoninus. How do we know if a physician is competent? Some claim that degrees from a university are a proof of competence. (Think of every doctor's office you have ever been in with the diplomas hanging on the wall.) But Antoninus realistically points out that there are many people in universities, both students and professors, who are not competent. For him the best criterion of competence is judgment by one's peers.[1]

Casuistry played a significant role in Catholic moral theology as Professors Jonsen and Toulmin have pointed out (Jonsen and Toulmin 1988, 137–26). Casuistry often became a pejorative term because some casuists, who became known as laxists, used casuistry to weaken or avoid moral obligation. One moral theologian was ironically described as "the lamb of God who takes away the sin of the world"! However, at its best, casuistry is a helpful and creative way of perceiving and trying to solve moral problems, as illustrated in the case of care for the dying.

Early on, the Catholic moral tradition had come to the conclusion that human beings do not have to do everything possible to keep human life in existence, based on the recognition that positive obligations can often conflict with other positive obligations. As a result, the tradition maintained that one has to use ordinary means but not extraordinary means to preserve life. A very widely accepted understanding of extraordinary means describes these as all medicines, treatments, and operations that cannot be obtained or used without excessive expense, pain, or other inconvenience, or that, if used, would not offer a reasonable hope of benefit (Kelly 1958, 129). In the light of developing technology, the major problem faced in the middle of the twentieth century concerned the continued use of means such as the respirator or the nasogastric tube that would only prolong the dying process and not offer any reasonable hope of success. For many this seemed to be a new question. However, in the seventeenth century, the casuist Juan de Lugo creatively raised the issue of no hope of success or benefit with an imaginative case. A person condemned to death by burning at the stake can manage to get some water to douse the flames and prolong his life. But there is no obligation to do so because the captors will just light the fire again (Cronin 1958, 64). Here one sees the best of creative casuistry at work imagining a problem that only became quite prominent with the development of modern technology.

In addition to the significant ethical dimension, the Roman Catholic tradition had other reasons for staying in contact with developing medical and biological sciences. Catholic canon law dealt with many aspects of life, including the laws governing marriage. To enter marriage, a couple had to be able to perform the marital act. The tradition thus recognized the distinction between impotency (the inability of the couple to perform the marital act) and sterility (the inability to have children). This important distinction called for Catholic canonists to be conversant with the medical knowledge of the time to determine the difference between impotency and sterility (Antonelli 1901). Beginning in 1621, Paolo Zacchia published a multivolume work, *Quaestiones medico-legales*, dealing with subjects impinging upon the relationship among medicine, law, and theology that became a standard reference book for Catholic moral theologians even as late as the nineteenth century (Zacchia 1701). Also in the seventeenth century, books appeared on the question of baptizing the fetus in the womb and on the morality of cesarean sections (Florentinus 1658; Raynaudus 1637). Franciscus Emmanuel Cangiamila's eighteenth-century book on sacred embryology was published in four different languages (Hurter 1962, 4:1646). In the nineteenth and twentieth centuries, a subdiscipline called pastoral medicine came into existence with the purpose of providing the priest with the medical knowledge needed to carry out his ministry and the doctor with the moral principles to insure that the doctor's actions are in accord with Christian morals (Capellmann 1879; Antonelli 1905; Niedermeyer 1948–52). In the United States, courses in medical ethics existed for nurses and doctors in Catholic colleges and universities, and textbooks were written for these courses as the twentieth century developed.[2] At the same time, the many addresses on medical moral issues by Pope Pius XII, who spoke not only to Catholics but often to international meetings of medical specialists in Rome, gave further impetus to Catholic interest in medical ethics.[3] All this explains why and how the Catholic tradition developed a strong interest in and concern for medical ethics long before 1960.

Two Other Questions

The second question naturally arises: Why were other Christian ethicists, philosophical ethicists, and legal scholars not interested in medical ethics before 1960? The primary reason is that there were not that many controversial issues, because for all practical purposes good medicine and good morality had the same basic criterion—what is for the good of the patient. Whatever is for the good of the patient is morally, medically, and legally good. Consequently, there were no real tensions between good medicine and good morality.

One major difference between Catholics and other approaches to marriage and medical morality before 1960 concerned the distinction between contraception and sterilization. Why did official Catholic teaching condemn direct sterilization while most others in society accepted it? The official Catholic teaching rested on the understanding that the sexual organs had a twofold purpose or finality—the good of the species and the good of the individual (Kelly 1958, 149–217). One could not subordinate the good of the species to the good of the individual. Most others rejected the absolute good of the species argument and justified contraception and sterilization if it were for the good of the individual or the marriage. Thus, the distinctive Catholic position on contraception and sterilization did not accept the criterion in this area that the moral good depends on what is good for the individual person. But in all other cases outside sexual issues, the Catholic position endorsed the moral criterion of what is for the good of the individual patient.

And the third question: Why the growth of bioethics since 1970? In many ways technology occasioned the great interest and growth in bioethics. First, technological developments made possible new realities that questioned the established criterion that good morality and good medicine depended on what was for the good of the patient. Transplants of paired organs such as kidneys became possible in the 1950s. Now, for the first time, medicine did harm to one patient in order to help another. Experimentation fueled the tremendous growth in medical procedures and drugs. The researcher as such was not primarily interested in the good of the individual patient, but rather the good of science and the knowledge that could be used to help others in the future. Thus, the most fundamental principle of traditional medical ethics—do no harm to the patient— no longer held.

Technology developed significantly new ways of bringing human life into existence whereas previously the only known process was the natural process of the sexual act. Even in the 1960s, people talked about the possibilities of cloning. Developments in genetics and technology raised a slew of new questions. These significant issues faced many people in their daily lives, and also became matters of legal interest and public policy. Technology thus constitutes the primary occasion for the tremendous development of bioethics since 1970.

MY PERSPECTIVE IN 1972

Vatican Council II (1962–65) introduced new understandings in Catholic thought and life. Catholic moral theology in general underwent significant developments after Vatican II. So significant were these developments that the leading Catholic moral theologians before Vatican II were not comfortable with the Vatican II approaches. I tried to approach moral theology and Catholic medical ethics and bioethics in the light of my understandings of the council.

The Shift to Historical Consciousness

Bernard Lonergan, the Canadian theologian who taught in Rome, pointed out that the primary change at Vatican II was the shift from classicism to historical consciousness. Classicism emphasized the eternal, the immutable, and the unchanging and employed a deductive methodology. Historical consciousness recognizes the subject, the historical, the particular, and the contingent, and employs a more inductive methodology (Lonergan 1967, 126–33). In my judgment a more inductive methodology recognizes that our understanding of anthropology is not something fixed forever but develops somewhat over time. Consequently, Catholic moral theology has to be open to learn some things about the human from all other interested perspectives and disciplines, including science and technology. In a sense, the relationship should be dialogical, but this does not mean that moral theology cannot and should not at times criticize the scientific and technological—a point I will develop later.

A more inductive approach can never claim the same certitude that the pre–Vatican II deductive Catholic moral theology claimed. The syllogism, the characteristic logical device of deduction, maintains that the conclusion is just as certain as the premises provided the logic is correct. A more inductive moral method has to be more tentative in its specific conclusions without, however, failing to take positions (Curran 1968, 109–53).

The Pastoral Constitution on the Church in the Modern World (Abbott 1966) employed a more historically conscious methodology by beginning its discussion of particular issues with an examination of the signs of the times. The classicist approach always began with the definition that was true at all times and in all places.

The best illustration of historical consciousness at work in the area of moral theology at Vatican II came from the Declaration on Religious Freedom. In this document the Catholic Church changed its teaching and recognized the universal right of all people to religious freedom. Discussions about this document in the council focused especially on how the church could change its teaching in this particular area. The generally accepted approach maintained that historical conditions had changed and the church in these new historical and cultural circumstances could now accept religious freedom for all (de Smedt 1964, 161–68). In my judgment the application of historical consciousness to explain this change too easily slid over the problem of the discontinuity between the earlier and the later teaching and the fact that there was error in the earlier teaching. But there can be no doubt that the methodology of the Declaration on Religious Freedom clearly illustrated historical consciousness at work.

In fact, Catholic social teaching in general had changed and developed with changing historical circumstances. In the nineteenth century the Catholic Church opposed liberalistic individualism with its emphasis on freedom, equality, and human rights. But as the twentieth century developed, the church turned its attention to the danger of totalitarianism, especially in the form of communism. Little by little, official Catholic social teaching began to defend human freedom, equality, and human rights (Murray 1965, 47–84). The Declaration on Religious Freedom well illustrated this change.

The obvious question arose: What effect would a more historically conscious methodology have in the area of Catholic sexual and medical ethics? I began to reexamine Catholic sexual and medical teaching in the light of this newer methodological approach.

A More Personalist Approach

The Pastoral Constitution on the Church in the Modern World (par. 51) proposes as the criterion for the harmonizing of conjugal love and the responsible transmission of life "the nature of the human person and his [sic] acts" (Abbott 1966, 256). The emphasis on the person was both new and important.

The Declaration on Religious Freedom (par. 1) begins by recognizing "a sense of the dignity of the human person has been imposing itself more and more deeply on the consciousness of contemporary man [sic]." Later the declaration (par. 2) affirms "that the right to religious freedom has its foundation in the very dignity of the human person" (Abbott 1966, 675, 679).

How would the criterion of the person affect Catholic sexual and medical ethics? Catholic moral theology had often insisted on the teleology of the God-given human faculties. The malice of lying well illustrates such an approach. The purpose of the faculty of speech is to put on my lips what is in my mind. In lying, the individual goes against the God-given purpose of the faculty of speech. Lying is defined as speaking something contrary to what is in the mind (Zalba 1952, 102–13). Catholic sexual ethics applied the same criterion of the teleology of the faculty to questions of sexuality. In this light, every act of the sexual faculty has to be both open to procreation and to love union, since these are the two God-given purposes of the sexual faculty (Zalba 1952, 324–26).

Some Catholic theologians even early in the twentieth century had abandoned the older faculty teleology approach to lying for a more personalist and relational criterion. The ultimate malice of lying does not consist in going against the God-given teleology of the faculty of speech but rather in the violation of the neighbor's right to truth. If the neighbor does not have the right to truth, then what one says may be false speech but this does not entail the moral malice of lying (Dorszynski 1949). It was only natural that in the light of the criterion of the person, Catholic moral theologians would also call into question the criterion of the teleology of the sexual faculty for determining what is morally right or wrong.[4]

Philosophical anthropology, intimately related to historical consciousness and personalism, came to the fore in the 1960s debate over artificial contraception. Those who disagreed with the official hierarchical teaching often criticized the official anthropology as suffering from physicalism. Physicalism identifies the human moral act with the physical aspect or structure of the act. In most cases Catholic moral theology avoids physicalism. Thus, killing, the physical act, is not always wrong. But in sexual ethics the physical act of the depositing of male semen in the vagina of the female is sacrosanct and can never be interfered with. This physicalism explains not only the hierarchical opposition to artificial contraception but also to artificial insemination with the husband's sperm (AIH), to say nothing of artificial insemination with a donor's sperm (AID). Yes, the physical aspect is important, but it is only one aspect of the human and at times might be sacrificed for the good of the total human. I also challenged other areas of Catholic moral theology in which the physical was identified with the moral, such as in the third principle of the double effect that calls for the good effect not to be caused by means of the evil effect, and the doctrine that human life begins from the very moment of conception (Curran 1969, 159–67).

An adequate anthropology thus recognizes that the human is the ultimate aspect that brings together all the partial aspects such as the physical, the psychological, the sociological, the medical, the eugenic, the hygienic, etc. Such an anthropology recognizes the scientific and technological aspects as just one part of the human. The technological or scientific is basically good but limited. Hence, the fully human at times must say no to the technological. One thus cannot simply identify technological progress with human progress. At times the human should and must say no to the absolutization of the technological that is not bad but is a limited good that must be relativized in the light of the fully human.

The Ecumenical Dialogue

Vatican II, especially in its Decree on Ecumenism, recognized the importance of dialogue with other Christian churches. In the pre–Vatican II period, hostility rather than dialogue characterized the Catholic approach to other religions—even Christian religions. The presence of Protestant observers at the Second Vatican Council, and the role they played in the council, illustrated the importance of ecumenical dialogue in the renewal of the life of the Catholic Church.

Catholic theology before the Second Vatican Council had practically no dialogue whatsoever with Protestant thought but tended to treat Protestants as the adversaries who had to be refuted. In 1972, at the Kennedy Institute, I decided to write a monograph on the political and medical ethics of Paul Ramsey, the leading Protestant ethicist in the United States at that time. Ramsey, in the late 1960s, had entered wholeheartedly into the area of medical ethics and bioethics with in-depth discussions on various aspects including genetics.[5] Without doubt, many Catholic theologians, including myself, learned much from Ramsey, but, at the same time, I pointed out significant methodological differences between Ramsey's approach and my own approach out of the Catholic tradition. In some ways this was a pioneering work in the early 1970s, but later on all Catholic moral theology became ecumenical, so that one could no longer do Catholic moral theology without bringing in the ecumenical dimension.

The Renewal of Moral Theology

Vatican Council II, especially in its Decree on Priestly Formation (par. 16), called for the renewal of moral theology with a greater emphasis on its Scriptural and theological aspects. Pre–Vatican II moral theology was based almost exclusively on human nature and human reason. The realm of the supernatural rested on top of the natural but did not directly affect it. The emphasis of Vatican II and my work on Ramsey helped me to focus more on the theological aspects of the discipline of moral theology. Eschatology sees the world in relationship to the fullness of the reign of God. Ramsey's apocalyptic eschatology is one-sided. An apocalyptic eschatology sees an oppositional or, at best, paradoxical relationship between the divine and the human. God's power is made known in human weakness; joy in sorrow, death in life. A more balanced eschatology, in my judgment, should recognize some continuity between the now and the then. God's love is also present in human love and God's beauty in created beauty. The traditional Roman Catholic emphasis on mediation has always seen the divine as also working in and through the human (Curran 1973, 200–205).

Eschatology obviously relates to theological anthropology. In any approach to bioethics, much depends on whether one is optimistic or pessimistic about the human project. Ramsey, in my judgment, is too pessimistic. I developed what I call the stance of moral theology—the perspective from which the discipline looks at the world. The Christian looks at the world on the basis of the fivefold stance of creation, sin, incarnation, redemption, and resurrection destiny. Creation recognizes the goodness of all God has made; sin affects creation but does not totally destroy it and is not the last word; incarnation recognizes the basic goodness of the human since God became human; redemption grounds the existence of God's grace already present and working in the world, but resurrection destiny as the future of the reign of God recognizes that the fullness of God's grace and reign will only come at the end of time. Such a stance by definition opposes a one-sided theological anthropology that overemphasizes either pessimism or optimism (Curran 1970, 85–110).

The Theological Aspect of Moral Theology

In the post–Vatican II Catholic Church, the 1968 encyclical *Humanae Vitae* reiterated the condemnation of artificial contraception and raised the question about the legitimacy of dissent both in theory and in practice from authoritative noninfallible hierarchical teaching. For many reasons I recognize the possibility and need for such dissent. By its very nature, teaching on specific moral issues is not that directly connected to matters of faith. In fact, the very description of such teaching as noninfallible recognizes that it is fallible and therefore might be wrong. The earlier insistence on a more inductive methodology also argues against the absolute certitude that had too often been connected with conclusions in Catholic moral theology before Vatican II (Curran 1986).

The Catholic tradition has long recognized the difficulty in claiming absolute certitude as one moves from the general to the particular and the specific, precisely because more circumstances are involved on the specific level. Without doubt a serious tension exists between the two most significant sources of specific Catholic moral teaching—human reason and the authoritative teaching office of the church. The authoritative teaching office always claimed that its teachings were based on human reason but that, in the process of formulating the teaching, the hierarchical teaching office had the assistance of the Holy Spirit. I emphasize, however, that the assistance of the Holy Spirit does not do away with the need for all the human processes of trying to arrive at moral wisdom and truth, but helps in this process. The traditional Thomistic teaching long ago raised the question: Is something good because it is commanded or is it commanded because it is good? The response of Thomas Aquinas clearly insisted on an intrinsic morality that something is commanded because it is good. Not all Catholic moral theologians agree with the possibility and need for such dissent, and to this day the hierarchical magisterium has taken disciplinary action against some who dissent and has never positively affirmed the legitimacy of such dissent. Thus, this tension between authoritative teaching and human reason continues to exist in Roman Catholicism.

Significant continuity, however, exists between pre–Vatican II and post–Vatican II moral theology. The Catholic tradition insists on being catholic, universal, and inclusive. "Both-and" rather than "either-or" approaches tend to characterize Catholic positions as illustrated in the understandings of eschatology and anthropology mentioned above. Catholic theology has always seen the divine as mediated in and through the human. The human and human reason are consequently good but limited and subject to sin. Post–Vatican II moral theology continues to give a prominent role to human reason and, in the light of a more inductive approach, human experience. The Catholic tradition of casuistry remains an important but only a partial aspect of moral theology (Curran 1999, 1–59). In my judgment, Richard A. McCormick, the most significant Catholic bioethicist in the latter part of the twentieth century, was primarily a casuist who incorporated Vatican II understandings into his approach. This section thus explains the approach that I took to doing bioethics in the early 1970s.[6]

LOOKING BACKWARD AND FORWARD FROM TODAY

The discipline of bioethics has grown immensely since 1971. Newer questions arise almost every day. The discipline now recognizes many different perspectives—the physician, the nurse, the patient, and the health care institution. Bioethics touches on many disciplines—philosophy, theology, law, political science. The move away from an exclusive quandary ethics has led to a place for virtue ethics and especially considerations of social aspects such as the distribution of health care. Since Catholic bioethics has also experienced many developments, the following brief observations do not pretend to be comprehensive or exhaustive.

A Backward Glance

With regard to Catholic bioethics, the complexity of the issues and the breadth of the discipline mean that one has to specialize in bioethics and cannot be a generalist in moral theology covering all the different areas of the discipline. In the light of this situation, I personally decided in the late 1970s to move out of bioethics and to concentrate more in other areas. Current scholars in Catholic bioethics, with one or two exceptions, tend to specialize primarily in bioethics. The very complexity of the discipline calls for such specialization, and specialization will be even more necessary in the future with the continuing growth of bioethics.

The differences within Catholic bioethics have hardened considerably since 1971. On a theoretical plane, three generic approaches exist. The older neoscholastic approach that served as the basis of the hierarchical teaching; a new natural-law approach associated with Germain Grisez and John Finnis that strongly supports the positions of the hierarchical magisterium (Biggar and Black 2000); and a revisionist perspective that disagrees with and dissents from some teachings of the hierarchical magisterium. This revisionist position is not monolithic but includes a variety of positions. The revisionist position today is regularly excluded from Catholic journals and institutes with some connection to the institutional church. For example, the *Linacre Quarterly* is the publication of the Catholic Medical Association. In the 1970s, revisionist bioethicists were members of the editorial advisory board and often published in the journal. But since the 1980s, Catholic revisionist bioethicists no longer serve on the advisory board, and the journal does not publish articles that disagree with the teaching of the hierarchical magisterium.[7] *Health Progress*, formerly called *Hospital Progress*, the official magazine of the Catholic Health Association, published revisionist articles in the 1970s, but lately no article appears that disagrees in any way with official teaching. The Religious and Ethical Directives for Catholic Health Care Services, the official code for Catholic health care institutions, have been even more restrictive lately in their interpretation of hierarchical teaching.[8] The National Catholic Bioethics Center, which began in 1972 as the Pope John XXIII Medico-

Moral Research and Education Center, has no place today in its publications and workshops for positions disagreeing with any existing hierarchical teaching (www.ncbcenter.org). Thus, no dialogue takes place today in these journals and publications.

At the present time, Catholic hospitals in accord with the ethical directives cannot cooperate in any way with sterilizations. This position has also hardened over the past thirty years and shows no immediate signs of changing.

A Forward Glance
The primary tension within Catholic bioethics over the issue of dissent from hierarchical teaching will continue for the immediate future. Many of us hope that in the future official Catholic teaching will change on a number of these issues, but there are no signs of possible change on the horizon. Likewise, the differences and disagreements among Catholic bioethicists themselves will also not go away. However, divisions and differences among Catholic bioethicists tend to be less in the areas of bioethics that are receiving more attention today—for example, virtue ethics, and the social aspect of medicine dealing with the just and proper distribution of health care in society.

Much has been written about the fact that religious ethics today plays a much-reduced role in bioethics. One illustration of this is the centuries-old understanding concerning ordinary and extraordinary means for preserving life, mentioned earlier. Paul Ramsey referred to this as the "oldest morality there is . . . concerning responsibility toward the dying" (Ramsey 1998, 224). He had studied the Catholic tradition in some depth and developed his own approach in the light of it. The November–December 2001 issue of the *Hastings Center Report* has only the following words on the cover: "End of Life Care: The Forgotten Catholic Tradition" (Panicola 2001, 14–25).

This is not the place to review and evaluate the literature that exists on the marginalization of religious bioethics and what might and should be done about it, but one comment is in order. Within Christian bioethics today, two different approaches exist. Some claim that Christian bioethics should directly address only the Christian community and not the broader human community in general or the aspects of law and public policy (Hauerwas 1990). A second position maintains that Christian ethics addresses two different audiences—the church and the broader human community. Again, a full discussion of these two positions lies beyond the parameters of this essay, but one point deserves mentioning. The Catholic tradition with its emphasis on mediation, the human, inclusiveness, and universality has always had a concern for what takes place in the world and has tried to address such issues. Recall the two pastoral letters on peace and the economy written by the U.S. Catholic bishops in the 1980s and addressed to both the church and the broader human society. The problems connected with this approach from Constantinianism to the present are well known, but the Catholic tradition to be true to itself must continue to address both the church and the world (Curran 1999, 1–29).

In the future the official Catholic approach to law and public policy must become more conscious of the difference between law or public policy and morality—as the distinction was developed in the Declaration on Religious Freedom of Vatican II. Too often, official Catholic statements move from morality immediately to legality or policy. But the Declaration on Religious Freedom proposed a more nuanced approach to the relationship between law or public policy and morality.

The declaration (par. 7) accepted the fundamental principle of a free society—as much freedom as possible and as little restraint as necessary. The document proposes public order as the criterion to justify and require the intervention of the state. According to Vatican II, public order embraces the goods of justice, public peace, and public morality.

In the light of this approach, the following three principles govern the justification of the coercive use of law in a pluralistic society: (1) As much freedom as possible and as little restraint as necessary; (2) Law can and should intervene to preserve and promote justice, public peace, and public morality; and (3) There is a pragmatic aspect to all laws. Is the law feasible? Can it be passed? Can it be enforced? Often legislators will be forced to compromise in order to get a law passed that in their judgment is somewhat imperfect but better than nothing. This understanding of law recognizes some pragmatic aspects but, at the same time, also does not reduce law only to the pragmatic—as illustrated in the second principle calling for law to protect and promote justice, public peace, and public morality.

In the United States in the last thirty years, the Roman Catholic Church has strenuously attempted to support laws prohibiting abortion (Byrnes and Segers 1992). How does the foregoing approach to civil law relate to the question of whether or not there should be a law against abortion? In this analysis I will presume the official Catholic teaching that direct abortion is morally wrong. One could justify supporting abortion legislation on the basis of the principles described above by invoking especially the second principle, that law should intervene to protect justice. If one believes that the fetus is a truly human person, then justice demands there be a law to protect the life of the fetus.

On the other hand, one could use the first and third principles in the approach mentioned above to come to the conclusion that there should be no law against abortion in our pluralistic society today. On the basis of the first principle—as much freedom as possible and as little restraint as necessary—one can argue that the present divisions and impasse in this country over abortion mean that the freedom of people who believe in the possibility of abortion should be respected. When the civil society is heavily divided, the presumption is in favor of freedom. Likewise the pragmatic aspects of the above theory of law could argue against an abortion law. Many have pointed out (but not without rebuttal) that laws condemning abortion would ultimately be unenforceable. Above all, pragmatic aspects of feasibility come to the fore. There does not seem to be the possibility of passing such laws at the present time.

In the light of the Vatican II approach, the primary way for the church to affect society is not through the coercive force of law but by freely entering the public dialogue and trying to convince others by the church's own elaboration of and witness to the truth.[9] In my judgment, the pastoral letters of the U.S. bishops on peace and the economy followed this approach and as a result played a significant role in the public debate over these issues in the United States.

There is no doubt that there will continue to be acrimonious debates in our society about public policy and laws dealing with questions of bioethics. From the viewpoint of theology, I believe Christian churches, including the Catholic Church, have a right to speak up on these issues and to work for appropriate public policy. However, in so doing, I think the Catholic Church must become much more conscious of the approach to law and morality that was proposed at the Second Vatican Council but often has not been mentioned in the discussion about law and public policy in the United States in the last thirty years.[10] At the very minimum, this approach does not rely only or primarily on law; it recognizes more ambiguity about the role of law than official Catholic statements recognize.

I have tried to show how I approach bioethics in the light of the Catholic tradition while recognizing that there are other, different approaches within that tradition. No one can accurately predict what developments will occur as the Catholic moral tradition addresses bioethics in the future, but the church must continue to speak publicly to these issues.

NOTES

1. See also Florentini 1740; Vereecke 1986, 259–82.

2. See the books published in the United States, including Healy 1956; Kelly 1958; Kenny 1952; and O'Donnell 1956.

3. Kenny (1962, 272) lists in his index forty topics in medical ethics that Pope Pius XII addressed.

4. For an early (1928) criticism of the faculty teleology argument in sexuality in the light of the changed approach to lying, see Ryan 1999, 120–23. But Ryan still held to the condemnation of artificial contraception (1999, 132–34). In a recent development, Cardinal Joseph Ratzinger promulgated final changes in the Catechism of the Catholic Church which "corrected" the previous teaching of the catechism that explicitly saw the malice of lying in light of the violation of the neighbor's right to truth. (Ratzinger 1997, 262).

5. Paul Ramsey's books on bioethics include Ramsey 1970a, 1970b, 1975, and 1978.

6. For an overview and analysis of McCormick's work, see Odozor 1995.

7. Recently a Catholic ethicist who is identified more with a revisionist approach published an article in the *Linacre Quarterly*, but the article itself did not disagree with any hierarchical teachings; see Walter 2001, 319–34.

8. For the latest edition of these directives (2001), see www.nccbuscc.org/bishops/directives.htm (accessed March 10, 2003).

9. Hermínio Rico (2002) distinguishes this approach, which he sees as grounded in Vatican II, from the approach taken by Pope John Paul II.

10. For essays from various positions on the role of the U.S. Catholic bishops in law and public policy, see Curran and Griffin 2002, 141–247, 291–310. For one bishop who employed the criterion about the relationship between morality and law as developed in the Declaration on Religious Freedom, see Joseph L. Bernardin's article in Curran and Griffin 2002, 160–69.

REFERENCES

Abbott, Walter M. 1966. Pastoral Constitution on the Church in the Modern World. In *The Documents of Vatican II*. New York: Association.

Antonelli, Josephus. 1901. *Pro conceptu impotentiae et sterilitatis relate ad matrimonium*. Rome: Pustet.

——. 1905. *Medicina pastoralis*. 2 vols. Rome: Pustet.

Bernardin, Joseph L. 2002. Consistent Ethic of Life. In *The Catholic Church, Morality, and Politics: Readings in Moral Theology No. 12*, edited by C. E. Curran and L. Griffin. New York: Paulist Press.

Biggar, Nigel, and Rufus Black, eds. 2000. *The Renewal of Natural Law: Philosophical, Theological, and Ethical Responses to the Finnis-Grisez School*. Burlington, Vt.: Ashgate.

Bonnar, Alphonsus. 1939. *The Catholic Doctor*. 2d ed. London: Burns, Oates.

Byrnes, Timothy A., and Mary C. Segers, eds. 1992. *The Catholic Church and the Politics of Abortion: A View from the States.* Boulder, Colo.: Westview.

Cangiamila, Emmanuel. 1766. *Abregé de l'Embryologie sacrée.* 2d ed. Paris: Nyon.

Capellmann, Carolus. 1879. *Medicina pastoralis.* 7th ed. Aquisgrani: R. Barth.

Cronin, Daniel A. 1958. *The Moral Law in Respect to the Ordinary and Extraordinary Means of Conserving Life.* Rome: Pontificia Universitas Gregoriana.

Curran, Charles E. 1968. Absolute Norms and Medical Ethics. In *Absolutes in Moral Theology?* edited by C. E. Curran. Washington, D.C.: Corpus.

———. 1969. Natural Law and Contemporary Moral Theology. In *Contraception: Authority and Dissent,* edited by C. E. Curran. New York: Herder and Herder.

———. 1970. The Stance or Horizon of Moral Theology. In *The Pilgrim People: A Vision of Hope,* edited by J. Papin. Villanova, Penn.: Villanova University Press.

———. 1973. *Politics, Medicine, and Christian Ethics: A Dialogue with Paul Ramsey.* Philadelphia: Fortress.

———. 1986. *Faithful Dissent.* Kansas City, Mo.: Sheed and Ward.

———. 1999. *The Catholic Moral Tradition Today: A Synthesis.* Washington, D.C.: Georgetown University Press.

Curran, Charles E., and Leslie Griffin, eds. 2002. *The Catholic Church, Morality, and Politics: Readings in Moral Theology No. 12.* New York: Paulist Press.

de Smedt, Émile-Joseph. 1964. Religious Freedom. In *Council Speeches of Vatican II,* edited by Y. Congar, H. Küng, and D. O'Hanlon. London: Sheed and Ward.

Denzinger, Henricus, et al., eds. 1963. *Enchiridion symbolorum definitionum et declarationum de rebus fidei et morum.* 32d ed. Barcelona: Herder.

Dorszynski, Julius A. 1949. *Catholic Teaching about the Morality of Falsehood.* Washington, D.C.: Catholic University of America Press.

Florentini, Sanctus Antonius Archiepiscopus. 1740. *Summa, pars tertia.* Verona: Typographia Seminarii.

Florentinus, Girolamo. 1658. *De hominibus dubiis baptizandis.* Lyon.

Hauerwas, Stanley. 1990. *Naming the Silences: God, Medicine, and the Problem of Suffering.* Grand Rapids, Mich.: William B. Eerdmans.

Healy, Edwin F. 1956. *Medical Ethics.* Chicago: Loyola University Press.

Hurter, Hugo. 1962. *Nomenclator literarius theologiae catholicae theologos exhibens aetate, natione, disciplinis distinctos.* Vol. 4. New York: B. Franklin.

Jonsen, Albert R., and Stephen Toulmin. 1988. *The Abuse of Casuistry: A History of Moral Reasoning.* Berkeley: University of California Press.

Kelly, Gerald. 1958. *Medico-Moral Problems.* St. Louis: Catholic Hospital Association.

Kenny, John P. 1952. *Principles of Medical Ethics.* Westminster, Md.: Newman.

———. 1962. *Principles of Medical Ethics.* 2d ed. Westminster, Md.: Newman.

Lonergan, Bernard. 1967. A Transition from a Classicist Worldview to Historical Mindedness. In *Law for Liberty: The Role of Law in the Church Today,* edited by J. E. Biechler. Baltimore: Helicon.

Murray, John Courtney. 1965. *The Problem of Religious Freedom.* Westminster, Md.: Newman.

Niedermeyer, Albert. 1935. *Pastoralmedizinische propädeutik.* Salzburg: Pustet.

———. 1948–52. *Handbuch der speziellen pastoral-medizin.* 6 vols. Vienna: Herder.

O'Donnell, Thomas J. 1956. *Morals in Medicine.* Westminster, Md.: Newman.

Odozor, Paulinus Ikechukwu. 1995. *Richard A. McCormick and the Renewal of Moral Theology.* Notre Dame, Ind.: University of Notre Dame Press.

Panicola, Michael. 2001. Catholic Teaching on Prolonging Life: Setting the Record Straight. *Hastings Center Report* 31, no. 6 (November–December): 14–25.

Paquin, Jules. 1957. *Morale et médecine.* 2d ed. Montréal: Immaculée Conception.

Payen, P. G. 1935. *Déontologie médicale d'après le droit naturel.* Zi-Ka-Wei: T'ou-se-we.

Pujiula, Jacobus. 1953. *De medicina pastorali.* 2d ed. Turin: Marietti.

Ramsey, Paul. 1970a. *Fabricated Man: The Ethics of Genetic Control.* New Haven, Conn.: Yale University Press.

———. 1970b. *The Patient as Person: Explorations in Medical Ethics.* New Haven, Conn.: Yale University Press.

———. 1975. *The Ethics of Fetal Research.* New Haven, Conn.: Yale University Press.

———. 1978. *Ethics at the Edges of Life.* New Haven, Conn.: Yale University Press.

———. 1998. The Indignity of "Death with Dignity." In *On Moral Medicine: Theological Perspectives in Medical Ethics,* edited by S. E. Lammers and A. Verhey. Grand Rapids, Mich.: William B. Eerdmans.

Ratzinger, Cardinal Joseph. 1997. Vatican List of Catechism Changes. *Origins* 27.

Raynaudus, Theophilus. 1637. *De ortu infantium.* Lyons.

Rico, Hermínio. 2002. *John Paul II and the Legacy of Dignitatis Humanae.* Washington, D.C.: Georgetown University Press.

Ryan, John A. 1999. Birth Control: The Perverted Faculty Argument. In *The Historical Development of Fundamental Moral Theology in the United States: Readings in Moral Theology No. 11,* edited by C. E. Curran and R. A. McCormick. New York: Paulist Press.

Scremin, Luigi. 1953. *Dizionario di morale professionale per i medici.* 5th ed. Rome: Editrice Studium.

Vereecke, Louis. 1986. Médecine et morale chez saint Antonin de Florence. In *De Guillaume d'Ockham à Saint Alphonse de Liguori: Études d'historie de la théologie morale moderne 1300–1787.* Rome: Collegium S. Alfonsi de Urbe.

Walter, James J. 2001. Human Gene Transfer: Some Theological Contributions to the Ethical Debate. *Linacre Quarterly:* 319–34.

Zacchia, Paolo. 1701. *Quaestiones medico-legales.* 3 vols. Lyons: Posuel.

Zalba, Marcellinus. 1952. *Teologia Moralis Summa.* Vol. 3. Madrid: Biblioteca de autores cristianos.

7

Richard A. McCormick, S.J.'s
"To Save or Let Die: The Dilemma
of Modern Medicine"

LISA SOWLE CAHILL

R ichard McCormick was one of the twentieth century's leading
Catholic theologians. He made many important contributions
to bioethics, especially in the "Notes on Moral Theology" he
authored in *Theological Studies* for over twenty years, which were eagerly
awaited every March by Catholic theologians and pastors. Since Dick left
this world only three years ago, it is not inappropriate to linger for a
moment on an elegiac note. Here are some words his good friend, colleague, coauthor, and co-conspirator, Charles Curran, delivered on the
occasion of Dick's funeral. "Dick skillfully wove together common sense,
perceptive analysis, a critical intelligence, and an ability to cut through
the debate to the salient feature of a problem. McCormick possessed to
an eminent degree the virtues of a good moral theologian. He was a
judicious, objective, calm, well-balanced observer who needed to be convinced by rational arguments. However, he was not unduly hesitant to
decide issues and always had the courage of his conviction."

McCormick in Context

These good qualities are perfectly illustrated in the short article, now
almost thirty years old, that the editors of this volume suggested I address.
The choice was an excellent one. "To Save or Let Die," a brief discussion
of allowing an infant to die, was published simultaneously in the *Journal
of the American Medical Association* and the Jesuit weekly *America* (Mc-
Cormick 1974). This fact in itself displays McCormick's aptitude for
speaking about ethics both in Catholic circles and to a larger public. The
genre, a semi-popular essay in which complicated or seemingly arcane

131

theological points are clarified in their relevance to current social debates, is one in which he excelled, though not the only one. In the mid-1970s, many social factors made care for the dying and critically ill a publicly visible, theologically timely, and medically (as well as legally) urgent topic. A pro-euthanasia movement was under way, receiving visible and vociferous advocacy from Derek Humphries and the Hemlock Society. Expanding possibilities for saving life in neonatal and adult intensive care units made the wisdom and expense of doing so worthy of attention. In 1968 the so-called "Beecher Report" offered criteria for declaring still-breathing patients brain-dead, permitting the removal of useful organs (Beecher 1968). Meanwhile, other theologians, such as McCormick's Protestant colleagues Paul Ramsey and James Gustafson, were entering this fray and others that defined the opening of the era of modern bioethics.

In 1970, Ramsey had published *The Patient as Person*, in which he endorsed the new paradigm of "brain death." He also used the traditional Catholic distinction between ordinary and extraordinary means of life support (see Kelly 1957, 129) to argue that efforts to save life have proper limits, limits that he judged to have been met when prolonging life turns into a " 'war' . . . against God for the last shred of sentient life" (Ramsey 1970, 119). At this point the duty is to "only" care for the admittedly dying person. Ramsey also hinted, barely, that when severe pain is unavoidable, some more direct action might be taken to end life (Ramsey 1970, 162). Gustafson, in turn, had written an essay replying to a notorious case at Johns Hopkins Hospital, in which parents had declined life-saving surgery for a newborn boy with Down's syndrome, on the grounds that the medical and psychosocial burdens of raising such a child were insupportable. While by no means laying down hard and fast rules about such decisions, Gustafson offered that it ought to be the child who is the center of the decision, and that it is far from clear that a person with Down's syndrome cannot lead a meaningful life (Gustafson 1973).

McCormick assessed these and other opinions on these questions in his "Notes on Moral Theology" covering works of 1972 (McCormick 1981b, 435–47).[1] He opened with this observation: "The over-all care for the dying has surfaced as a concern of much recent literature. I say 'surfaced' because this subject has been for too long a contemporary form of pornography: on everybody's mind but repressed from our cultural consciousness by every myth, taboo, and ritual we can bend to this purpose" (1981b, 435). McCormick then proceeded to lay out and debate the views of Arthur Dyck against euthanasia, and of Merle Longwood, Daniel Maguire, Joseph Fletcher, and Paul Ramsey in favor, albeit in very restricted circumstances. While a useful and not too onerous means of prolonging life may be considered mandatory, a useless or very burdensome means is not, and may be refused, preferably by the patient himself or herself, allowing for proxy decision making when necessary. McCormick conceded that the distinction between acts of omission and commission may not always be morally decisive. But he hesitated to go along with a final defense of directly killing even suffering and dying patients. With the Catholic tradition on ordinary and extraordinary means of life support, McCormick always maintained that withholding or withdrawing life supports is one thing, direct killing significantly another. Interestingly, McCormick conceded that a sort of intuitive sense of good moral-line-drawing may be the decisive factor in distinguishing and in holding the line against direct euthanasia. "Perhaps a concrete prohibition like the one in question [of mercy-killing] cannot be 'proved,' but it might well be the conclusion of prudence in the face of dangers too momentous to allow the matter to the uncertainties and vulnerabilities of individual decision" (1981b, 442–43). Behind this conclusion is a mistrust of our cultural acceptance of the pursuit of unlimited technological prowess, a skepticism McCormick said he shared with Daniel Callahan, and which Callahan continues to promote (see, for example, Callahan 1993).

As a context for "To Save or Let Die," this discussion highlights several important and typical characteristics of McCormick's approach to morality. First of all, his religious sensibilities were in evidence, but in the background. Among them I detect at least four: a respect for life and reticence toward its destruction; the relativization of the value of human life in light of interpersonal and spiritual values like care; a certain acceptance of some suffering as part of the human condition—to be avoided when reasonably possible, but not at all costs; and a sensitivity to the role of multiple values in decision making, some of which transcend mere logic. Second, McCormick both employed and reshaped the tools of Catholic moral theology, such as the distinction between ordinary and extraordinary means, the difference between direct and indirect action and intention, and the principle of totality. While reasonableness was his watchword, whether mediating disputes in the church or appealing to a broader audience of medical professionals and lawmakers, he stayed far away from the arid, syllogistic reason of some then-prevalent types of natural-law moral theology. He was willing to acknowledge that his argument is not always a clincher, but, as Curran said of him, he never lacked the courage of his convictions. "To Save or Let Die," in clarifying the reasons why it *is* acceptable sometimes to refrain from saving physical life, also helps elucidate why the line between direct and indirect killing is one that it is best not to cross.

"To Save or Let Die"

McCormick's article "To Save or Let Die" begins with a history of the short life and controversial death in 1974 of a baby boy at Maine Medical Center. The child had multiple deformities and almost surely was destined not to survive, or to survive only in a very grievously impaired state. Nevertheless, the Maine Superior Court ordered corrective surgery over the objections of the parents, on the grounds that the child was a human being with rights; the baby died not long thereafter. McCormick's basic response to this unhappy train of events was to defend the reasonableness of the parents' decision (in contrast to the Johns Hopkins case), and to do so by expressing in a clear and compelling way, and with a sense of immediacy, the wisdom of the Catholic moral tradition's past. Fundamental to his case is the argument that to affirm, as he does, that "every human being, regardless of age or condition, is of incalculable worth" does not imply that the lives of all should be indefinitely prolonged. The crux of McCormick's view is that it is precisely in light of human dignity that it makes sense to determine sometimes that continued life is not in the best interests of the patient himself or herself. Quality of life makes a difference. The highest value in human life, the one for which biological life is given, is love of God and neighbor. When life does not or can no longer serve as the condition for experiencing this "higher, more important good," then life has ceased to be a commanding value for the undoubtedly valued person. Death may be permitted to arrive, even by withdrawing technological measures that make it possible to go on (McCormick 1974, 176).

In arriving at his analysis, McCormick creatively and insightfully interprets sources from the recent Catholic tradition. First is the distinction between ordinary and extraordinary means, the latter being defined by the fact that "they involve grave hardships to the patients." A determination that they do is relative to the condition of the patient, and involves good judgment, not always certitude. McCormick also introduces the opinions of twentieth-century theologians (Gerald Kelly and M. Zalba) who, drawing on older traditions about the difficulty in obtaining or using exotic remedies, extended the category "extraordinary" to include the factor of "crushing" financial cost and hence hardship to oneself or one's family.

McCormick's key insight, however, is that the very purpose of life can be put at risk by serious illness and physical suffering even more than by death. He quotes a 1957 statement of Pius XII cautioning that "a more strict obligation" requiring the use of any means to prolong biological life "would be too burdensome for most men and would render the attainment of the higher, more important good too difficult. Life, death, all temporal activities are in fact subordinated to spiritual ends" (McCormick 1981a, 174; Pius XII 1957, 396). Quality of life can be a determinative consideration even when treatment can save life indefinitely. A life so reduced that it would permit the concentration of personal resources on nothing so much as survival and endurance would obstruct "the very possibility of growth in love of God and neighbor," putting something else in first place instead of Pius XII's "higher, more important good." What this higher good comes down to, as in the case of infants, is "relational potential," the capacity to experience human relationships, to know the love of others and return it. A child with mental and physical handicaps can still lead a meaningful, worthwhile life. But when all else in life is subordinated to the mere effort for survival, then that life is not worth living, *from the standpoint of* the valued but afflicted person (McCormick 1974, 174). The person always has value, but life may lose value for the person. In the case of infants or others unable to decide on their own behalf, the judgment, always risky and often imprecise, is best undertaken by the parents or family, in consultation with medical advisors.[2]

SOCIAL AND ETHICAL DEVELOPMENTS

The next several years were to bring further challenges to this framework, including the Karen Ann Quinlan case, several highly publicized court cases involving the withdrawal of artificial nutrition and hydration (see Barry 1989; Wildes 1996), the gradual legal acceptance of direct euthanasia in the Netherlands (see Shannon 2001), and a second-wave movement for physician-assisted suicide in the United States (see Manning 1998; Keenan 1998; Bresnahan 1998; Fuller 1997). Meanwhile, the Catholic Church was moving ahead with a variety of responses, including the 1980 Vatican Declaration on Euthanasia (Congregation for the Doctrine of the Faith 1980), and a revision of the U.S. Bishops' "Ethical and Religious Directives" for Catholic health care (National Conference of Catholic Bishops 1995). Greater ethical and social concern about the expense of high-tech health care also played increasingly into the picture of moral analysis of care for the dying (see Callahan 1998; National Conference of Catholic Bishops 1993). And at a more general and foundational level, the basic natural-law approach out of which McCormick always wrote came under increasing challenge philosophically and politically. This approach had already been revised by McCormick and others even before the Second Vatican Council, by giving the conception of human nature a "personalist" twist. This made for a more nuanced concept of human nature by referring to individuality, freedom, and intersubjectivity, but the confidence of most Catholic moral theologians in the concept's basic viability remained for the most part unshaken.

McCormick was never one to attempt the great theological or philosophical synthesis, or to raise basic questions about catholic Christian belief. He invariably, to the end of his life, took for granted, and plied his craft within the dialogue among teaching church, Catholic moral tradition, and culture. This dialogue had been the context of Vatican II and documents such as *Gaudium et Spes* and even *Humanae Vitae*. To McCormick and colleagues like Charles Curran, "historical consciousness" was a way of moving the natural-law tradition and its staple principles like double effect into a more flexible and pastorally sensitive mode. McCormick never would have so much as considered taking seriously the radical postmodern ideas that all foundations are socially determined and that all analysis is purely relative to power constructs. To the contrary, the basic premise of McCormick's moral theory was always the reasonableness of moral experience, its essential generalizability, and the possibility of defining and ranking with more or less accuracy the values basic to personal well-being and the common good.

Nonetheless, as one can see in "To Save or Let Die," McCormick had an early affinity for some of the correctives now prominent in current philosophical and theological approaches to ethics. He did not believe that moral conclusions could be reached and defended purely on the basis of logic; he believed, rather, that they emerged within a worldview, in which, for example, one did or did not give credibility to a transcendent realm of being, the relativity of human scientific prowess, the need to deal constructively with some ineliminable suffering, the social interdependence of all persons, and the priority of caring first of all for society's victims and losers. Further, although on one level, the natural-law tradition could be seen as affirming the knowability to all of basic values outside of revelation (thus removing the need to speak religiously in public), McCormick unembarrassedly used religious language in places like the *Journal of the American Medical Association* to illuminate the moral high ground and inspire all comers to take a broader perspective from a higher elevation of concern than that afforded by mere scientism, pragmatism, self-interest, or cost-effectiveness.

McCormick's subsequent writings continued to resist the trend toward direct euthanasia, and to affirm and refine the traditional distinction between ordinary and extraordinary means of life support as a useful way to think ethically about care for the dying and eventual acceptance of death, nuanced to the condition and prospects of each patient.[3] An extraordinary means is one that offers no benefit or offers it only at disproportionate cost, primarily measured in terms of patient welfare. The commitment of caregivers "to curing disease and preserving life . . . must be implemented within a healthy and realistic acknowledgment that we are mortal" (McCormick 1989, 365). When physical existence is absolutized, it amounts to "medical idolatry" and often results conversely in abandonment of the patient when curing or even significant alleviation of disease is no longer a medical possibility. McCormick's advice to physicians is "Don't see death as the ultimate enemy" (1989, 365).

In more recent commentaries, McCormick replied further to legal controversies over the physician's obligation to treat, or parents' prerogative to refrain from treating, newborns with grave mental as well as physical disabilities. Developing "To Save or Let Die," he expanded the criterion of relational capacity into four guidelines that could be extended to other patient classes: (1) life-saving interventions ought not be omitted because of burdens they impose on the family or others, who are owed health care and social support by larger social bodies; (2) even relatively significant mental handicap is not alone adequate reason for nontreatment; (3) life-sustaining interventions may be omitted in cases of excessive hardship for the patient, especially if combined with a poor prognosis; and (4) they can be omitted if the anticipated life span is brief and if it requires artificial feeding (McCormick 1984b, 121; McCormick and Paris 1983). As McCormick observes, such guidelines are an attempt to make concrete the relations of coalescent values and burdens, even if expressed in nonabsolute form. In this case, the rules "do not replace prudence" but are "simply attempts to provide some outlines of the areas in which prudence should operate" (McCormick 1983, 121).

This basic standard, of the worth of life to the patient faced with living it, can function generally, guiding cases of critically ill adults as well as of infants. The criterion in termination-of-treatment decisions should be "best interests," including some consideration of future quality of life. Following Edmund Pellegrino, McCormick added some dimensions to the meaning of best interests, particularly for patients who were once competent (McCormick 1984a, 115–16). The first component is "medical good," that is, a reasonable prognosis regarding the effects of medical intervention on a condition or disease process. The second is "patient preferences," based on the individual's life situation and value system, as previously indicated by the patient or as inferred by his or her proxy. The third is "the good of the human as human," a phrase referring to humanistic or philosophical values such as freedom, rationality, consciousness, and creativity. The last is "the good of last resort," the frame of reference that "gives life ultimate meaning." This will vary depending on a patient's religious and moral commitments and will affect perceptions of "best interests" at a fundamental level. Various religious traditions, for example, view differently the meaning of suffering or the value of preserving all life no matter what its condition. Thus, persons will not always agree in their judgments of best interests. Nonetheless, McCormick, as essentially a natural-law thinker, remained committed to the possibility of hammering out some consensus about best interests and quality of life.

The conviction was demonstrated in his attention to such court cases as Quinlan, Fox, Saikewicz, Conroy, Herbert, Brophy, and Cruzan. Quality-of-life evaluations will be necessary and not available directly on the basis of "objective" medical criteria, i.e., on the basis of physical condition alone. (For McCormick's disagreement with Paul Ramsey's "medical indications policy," see McCormick 1978.) McCormick urged that decisions regarding incompetent patients be premised on their welfare reasonably construed; that they be undertaken by the family if possible; and that they be hindered neither by the confusion of treatment refusal with homicide, nor by the absence of some prior indication of the patient's own wishes (McCormick and Veatch 1980; McCormick 1981b, 107–10). The danger of "living will" legislation lies precisely in its tendency to create the impression that signed, legally binding statements are a necessary precondition of refusal of useless treatment (McCormick and Hellegers 1977).

ARTIFICIAL NUTRITION AND HYDRATION

The question of withdrawing artificial nutrition and hydration was posed by the cases of Clarence Herbert, Paul Brophy, and Nancy Cruzan, all of whom were so sustained in the sort of deep coma inappropriately and pejoratively termed "persistent vegetative state." The question was posed in a slightly different manner by the case of Claire Conroy, similarly situated and severely demented, but not comatose. McCormick was sensitive to the belief of some (Daniel Callahan, with qualifications; Gilbert

Meilaender; Mark Siegler and Alan J. Weisbard; all cited in McCormick 1989, 377–78) that feeding by any method has great symbolic value. He cautioned against its cessation, especially for incompetent patients. Nonetheless, it can be in the best interests of some patients to have artificial feeding withdrawn. Such cases would arise when the procedures are "futile"; when the patient cannot in any meaningful way be said to "benefit" (for instance, in a "persistent vegetative state"); or when the negative effects on the patient's quality of life outweigh the benefits (McCormick 1989, 385).

McCormick used this discussion to address four central issues: the notion of a dying patient; the nature of artificial nutrition and hydration; the intention of death; and the burden-benefit calculus. A patient cannot be said to be "nonterminal" in any way that closes moral discussion about withdrawing artificial feeding simply because his or her life can be extended through the use of medical treatments. Some treatments may alleviate an underlying and otherwise fatal condition, but not all such treatments need be used. Transplants, artificial hearts, and dialysis all substitute for natural functions; but there is not the same moral obligation to use all these in all situations. McCormick finds that the so-called "difference between a dying and nondying patient" often "roots in a value judgment about whether we ought to use the available technology or not." He suggests that the appropriate value judgment depends on whether the treatment offers "a return to relatively normal health" and "ultimate independence from the technology" (McCormick 1989, 379).

Further, he remains unconvinced that the nature of artificial feeding is not "medical treatment" and so is not subject to such criteria. Again, artificial nutrition is a technology that replaces a natural function. More-over, death cannot be said to be the "direct" intention of withdrawal of artificial feeding, and thus forbidden as "suicide" or "murder," any more than omission of other medical treatments refused by or for other critically ill patients. The moral evaluation depends on what a given treatment can be expected to do for a given patient.

The heart of the issue is the last consideration, the evaluation of bene-fits. McCormick does not believe that life in a persistent vegetative state should be construed as a benefit or value to the one in such a state. Instead, the interdependence between a person's biological condition and his or her ability to pursue life's goal of relationship must be considered. Demonstrating that it remains important to him to locate this basically philosophical analysis of the value of life squarely within the parameters of Roman Catholic thought, McCormick concluded that "the abiding substance of the church's teaching . . . is found in a basic value judgment about the meaning of life and death, one that refuses to absolutize either." "Those who would count mere vegetative life a patient-benefit have, I believe, slipped their grasp on the heart of Catholic tradition in this matter" (McCormick 1989, 385)—and, one might add, on common sense about the purpose of life and the place of death at the end of it.

McCormick criticized the Cruzan decision, limited in applicability though it was to Missouri, because it seems to disallow any consideration of "quality of life" in allowing a decision when the patient has no clearly expressed prior wishes (McCormick 1990, 11). His own recommendation was the development of policies, with safeguards, which would guide decisions to discontinue treatments that no longer serve the holistic interests of the patient. He was persuaded that such policies would reflect the moral convictions of most people:

> For several years, I have asked audience after audience if they would want artificial nutrition and hydration were they irreversibly unconscious. With virtual unanimity the answer has been no. These people were saying that they did not regard continuing in that condition a benefit to them. (McCormick 1990, 12)

McCormick also regarded as morally acceptable the withdrawal of all artificial supports, for many of the same reasons, in cases like that of Claire Conroy, who was not in a deep coma. Forced feeding of the semiconscious elderly, often against their own efforts to remove tubes, can be dehumanizing. He did advise extreme caution in policy guidelines, lest the justifying "best interests" of the patient slide to social burden for others (McCormick 1989, 386). However, the "bedrock" teaching of Catholicism confirms human experience at this point. Physical existence is not an absolute value. The determination that life support is morally "extraordinary," and not necessary to continue, need not be carried by the excessiveness of one particular treatment but can be referred more generally to the condition of the whole life of the patient. The burden of striving to attain the purpose of life, or the impossibility of striving to attain it at all, is a sufficient reason to discontinue what have then become disproportionate means (McCormick and Paris 1987, 361).

MERCY KILLING

Consistently with Catholic tradition, McCormick never defended direct euthanasia or mercy killing, though, unlike magisterial teaching, he granted that an absolute distinction between direct and indirect killing might not be totally cogent. He still, however, regarded life as a "basic value," and maintained that the norm against directly dispatching even a terminal or dying patient has yet to be persuasively refuted (McCormick 1973). Although he incisively found fault with the assumptions, equations, and inferences of formidable pro-euthanasia philosophers like Peter Singer and James Rachels, McCormick acknowledged in the end that the distinction between acts of omission and acts of commission that similarly and deliberately bring about the result of death may not bear all the moral weight that moral theology and philosophy have traditionally placed on it. Hence, he conceded, the character of the problem is "extremely complex," and "the discussion is far from over." He believed the distinction to be of enduring usefulness, though he was "far from sure how we ought to analyze it." Finally, it may be that there are "mysterious dimensions to the last phase of life, dying," dimensions that escape "the neatness and tightness of our moral concepts and categories." "To think otherwise could easily be to attribute to rational analysis and argument powers they do not have" (McCormick 1981b, 612).

This may be an opportune place to add a comment on McCormick's reputation as a proponent of "proportionalism," a moral theory that does not bear all that directly on his approach to death and dying. "Proportionalism" started out as a term of abuse, directed at revisionist Catholic interpreters of the principle of double effect who claimed that certain absolute norms against specific moral actions did not hold water. These thinkers were rejected by the *magisterium* because they disputed moral teachings against categories of sexual conduct, especially birth control. The proportionalists maintained, in general, that the moral quality of an act could not be determined unless the context, circumstances, and intentions were taken into account. Criticizing standard interpretations of the principle of double effect, they asserted that one of its basic categories, the "intrinsically evil act," was not at all clearly defined, is full of inconsistencies in the application, and in any event could not be a sole determinant of morality, apart from understanding the context of any given action. Their adversaries maintained that there are some physical acts that can be defined as wrong, regardless of circumstances. But for proportionalists, the ultimate determinant of morality is the proportion of good over evil in an act considered as a whole (see McCormick 1973). The defenders of traditional morality answered that this is no better than consequentialism or utilitarianism, and that certain things have to be defined as immoral, no matter what the consequences. McCormick accepted the term proportionalist as a description of his own position, but whether he really meant by it what his accusers claimed is another matter.

The point here is that McCormick never disagreed with magisterial teaching on euthanasia; and the teaching about artificial nutrition and hydration that he did disagree with has never been proposed as binding for the whole church. He did not need proportionalism to defend withdrawal of extraordinary means of life support, including artificial nutrition and hydration. However, the personalist, social, and holistic moral sensibility behind the proportionalist critique of double effect is evident in McCormick's retrieval of Pius XII's insistence that the criterion of the morality of any decision to permit death to occur is the "higher, more important good," which is the purpose of life.

On the issue of mercy killing it is clear that McCormick adopted a generally "teleological" position, but not one that was narrowly consequentialist. The higher, more important end of human life is union with God, expressed and realized through love of neighbor. To adopt this purpose or end as the criterion of moral activity is to grant that more concrete and specific moral actions have to be judged in its light. McCormick believed that the refusal of treatment could be consistent with and even demanded by this higher end. In this he is no different from Catholic tradition. Yet even though a proportionalist analysis might logically yield the conclusion that life as a limited or premoral good could not compete for priority with moral goods such as love or spiritual growth, and in fact could be directly sacrificed in their favor, McCormick was never willing to say that life could be taken directly to protect the moral integrity or dignity of the person. His analytical framework and vocabulary might have suggested a different outcome. But his intuitive sense of the practical interplay of factors surrounding the actual social acceptance of medically sanctioned killing did not permit a more permissive conclusion. He never accepted mercy killing or physician-assisted suicide. Here we see prudence governing and checking the lengths to which reconstruction of the traditional system of norms might go, especially when life is at stake. And yet, the general thrust of his thought, raising moral vision from the individual act to the wholeness of the moral life and ultimately to its transcendent context, is very apparent in McCormick's placement of decisions about causing death against the horizon of that "higher, more important good."

McCormick recognized that weighing against direct euthanasia are not only considerations of the intrinsic morality of individual acts, but the possible short- and long-term effects of accepting acts of commission that result in death. The "presumption of a common and universal danger" is enough to establish at least a "virtually exceptionless" norm against it (McCormick 1974, 318–20). This is a social consideration that obviously moves beyond—though it does not necessarily make obsolete—the older Catholic approach that upholds the "individual's right to life" in any considerations of direct killing. McCormick responded to a hypothetical case study of a man who cooperated with his elderly father's wish to be killed directly (by suffocation), rather than face a prolonged death and unacceptable "helplessness" as a result of colon cancer, by seeing it as a failure of compassionate care. The causes are not limited to, nor do they even primarily consist in, the moral misguidedness of the agent, however. McCormick diagnosed a complicit cultural context that promotes assisted suicide. Contributing factors include an interventionist mentality, along with an implicit denial of mortality and refusal to let anyone die who can be saved—as long as they have health insurance, that is, and without regard for spiraling costs. Overused intensive care units that "resemble high-tech hospices" not only waste resources, they frighten many of the ill or elderly into taking action before they lose the opportunity to do so. Converging with these two factors is an absolutization of morality as personal autonomy and of dignity as productivity and independence. An ideal of the self-sufficient moral agent feeds into the unacceptability of dependency while making choice the only criterion of the means of escape. The social picture of responsibility and support recedes into the distant background, virtually being reduced to legal protection for choice, whether to demand and use resources, or to end illness and decline by ending life itself (McCormick 1997; see also McCormick 1994, 149–64).

SPIRITUALITY, HEALTH CARE, AND DYING

McCormick's concern with a good for human beings that is even greater than life and takes precedence over it suggests a dimension to health care that is especially apropos of a theological approach to bioethics: spirituality. Sometimes McCormick referred to this higher good as "the good of last resort," which he defined as "the good that gives life ultimate meaning." Observing that "many of us call this good God or Jesus Christ," he recognized that different religious traditions experience God differently, and that this can have an impact on moral convictions and practices—for example, the necessity of preserving life (McCormick 1989, 360; 1984a, 116). In *Health and Medicine in the Catholic Tradition* (1984a), McCormick outlined a fundamental Christian understanding of suffering and death, one that constitutes a distinctive spiritual approach to moral decision making in times of illness and to the confrontation with death itself. Although Christians do not glorify suffering, they do view it in the larger perspective of the redemptive process. Even when the meaning of suffering cannot be reduced or comprehended, it is faced with trust in God. Grave illness can be a time of identification with Christ, of grace, and of a sharing in the strength of resurrection life (McCormick 1984a, 116–18).

> Human suffering and death are an inescapable part of human life. However, through his own suffering and death Jesus has taught us that suffering and dying can be a means of inner transformation to deeper life as well as a redemptive prayer for others. Health care personnel should be trained and available to help patients find meaning in their experience of suffering and dying. (McCormick 1984a, 13)

Following the German theologian Karl Rahner, McCormick viewed spirituality as an orientation to God that develops over the course of one's whole life, and that both guides the discernment of moral choices and is expressed in those choices. Yet spirituality is not reducible to specific choices. The spiritual life is a life of friendship with God that unfolds over time as we reflect on God's word, participate in the Eucharist, and care for the needs of others. "Like any friendship, this one must be nourished and fostered with mutual conversation, exchange of gifts, moments of quiet, strenuous acts of protection and resistance and glorious celebrations" (McCormick 1994, 63). Spirituality makes special demands or takes on a special shape in time of illness, aging, or dying. The freedom to make and carry out choices through independent moral agency can diminish. The person arrives at a state of dependency that our culture and its ethos of medical care find very difficult to accept.

McCormick borrowed from Drew Christiansen, S.J., to develop a "theology of dependence." "Dependency is an opportunity, a call to let ourselves go, to open up to God, to cling in trust to a power beyond our control, to see more clearly than ever the source and end of life" (McCormick 1984a, 158). Dependence on others is part of the human condition, and ultimately a sign of our radical dependence on God. The disposition to accept unavoidable suffering and diminishment in a spirit of trust, and to recognize that not even the most powerful technologies can or should fend off death at all costs, is part of a spirituality that views the highest and most important good for humans as friendship with God, and that sees God as the ultimate source of human healing and redemption.

DECIDING DEATH AND SOCIAL ETHICS

In questions of death and dying, as in other biomedical concerns, sensitivity to social justice has in recent years become much more acute. In his later biomedical reflections, McCormick pushes further in the social direction, stressing the inevitability of human interdependence, so threatening to the Western view of the person as "autonomous individual." Demands for the right to control the time, place, and manner of one's own death require a corrective acceptance of dependency, as has been noted (McCormick 1989, 218–19). Another aspect of interdependence is the obligation to use and distribute resources fairly for the common good. McCormick raised questions about whether cutting-edge life-saving devices and technologies may be on a collision course with just use of health care resources, as well as threatening genuine patient welfare in at least some cases.

Considering the artificial heart as one example, McCormick raises some challenging questions. Will a given technology obscure more basic social needs? Will it "comfort the afflicted in their unspoken heterodoxy, 'If it can be fixed, why worry about the breakdown?' " Will it promote or undermine our efforts to deal societally with the elderly? What overall quality of life will it enable? If an exotic technology becomes more widely available, how will its economic accessibility for some affect our notions of justice and fairness for others? Does private financing of research on such options move us too far away from public scrutiny and control? "What is the impact of medicine's move to a business ethos on its self-concept, its practitioners, and its quality?" (McCormick 1989, 260). The moral character of even a technology that promises to prolong life or alleviate disease can no longer be resolved by a simple (and individualist) appeal to the dignity and worth of every life; nor to an equally simple interpretation of a physician's duty to do the utmost for every patient; much less to the right of researchers and investors to develop, market, and sell biotech products to consumers.

These social questions, of course, go back to a centuries-old tradition of limiting the use of treatments due to economic and even lifestyle considerations on the part of the patient at risk of death. Traditional authors mentioned obtaining expensive foods, submitting to surgical procedures in pre-anesthesia and pre-antiseptic days, or moving to more healthful but very distant climates. Discussion of contemporary parallels would not be limited to the effects on the patient and family, but would place those individuals, together with caregivers, in a social network in which the common good demands not only that goods of health be shared but that these be balanced off against other human and social goods. These apply not only in the local community or even the nation, but also in a rapidly expanding and highly inequitable social context. While Richard McCormick did not live to address the most recent and pressing issues of globalization, nor their bearing on the value and protection of life in a medical context, there is enduring wisdom in his reminder that there is a "higher, more important good" against which life and death decisions must be made, and in responsibility to which institutions that provide or deny the conditions of life should be structured.

I would like to conclude this review of McCormick's thought and influence in his own voice, since he has been subjected for a significant number of pages to an interpretation that he has had the opportunity neither to approve nor to correct. I will select some lines near the end of "To Save or Let Die" that will let Dick's voice be recalled to us in theological tones—which, I have no doubt, is the way he would want it to be.

"It is the pride of Judeo-Christian tradition that the weak and defenseless, the powerless and unwanted, those whose grasp of the goods of life is most fragile . . . are cherished and protected as our neighbor in greatest need. Any . . . guideline that forgets this is . . . profoundly at odds with the gospel," as well as "corrosive" of our very "humanity" (McCormick 1974, 176).

NOTES

1. McCormick published annual reviews of moral theology in the journal *Theological Studies* from 1965. These "notes" through 1980 are published in one volume (McCormick 1981b).

2. For other discussions of "To Save or Let Die," see McCartney 1990; and Odozor 1995, 130–36, both of whom borrow the title of the article to head their own discussions. For further treatments of these same themes by other authors, see Walter and Shannon 1990.

3. The following discussion of McCormick's writings after "To Save or Let Die" is based in part on Cahill 1993.

REFERENCES

Barry, Robert. 1989. Feeding the Comatose and the Common Good in the Catholic Tradition. *The Thomist* 53: 1–30.

Beecher, Henry K. 1968. A Definition of Irreversible Coma: Report of the Ad Hoc Committee of the Harvard Medical School to Examine the Definition of Brain Death. *Journal of the American Medical Association* 205: 337–40.

Bresnahan, James F. 1998. Palliative Care or Assisted Suicide? *America* 178: 16–21.

Cahill, Lisa Sowle. 1993. On Richard McCormick: Reason and Faith in Post–Vatican II Catholic Ethics. In *Theological Voices in Medical Ethics*, edited by Allen Verhey and Stephen E. Lammers. Grand Rapids: Eerdmans.

Callahan, Daniel. 1993. *The Troubled Dream of Life: In Search of a Peaceful Death*. New York: Simon and Schuster.

———. 1998. *False Hopes: Why America's Quest for Perfect Health Is a Recipe for Failure*. New York: Simon and Schuster.

Congregation for the Doctrine of the Faith. 1980. *Declaration on Euthanasia*. Boston: St. Paul Editions.

Fuller, Jon. 1997. Physician-Assisted Suicide: An Unnecessary Crisis. *America* 177: 9–26.

Gustafson, James M. 1973. Mongolism, Parental Desires, and the Right to Life. *Perspectives in Biology and Medicine* 16: 529–59.

Keenan, James F. 1998. The Case for Physician-Assisted Suicide? *America* 179: 14–19.

Kelly, Gerald. 1957. *Medico-Moral Problems*. St. Louis: Catholic Hospital Association.

Manning, Michael. 1998. *Euthanasia and Physician-Assisted Suicide: Killing or Caring*? New York and Mahwah, N.J.: Paulist Press, 1998.

McCartney, James J. 1990. Issues in Death and Dying (Including Newborns). In *Moral Theology: Challenges for the Future*, edited by Charles E. Curran. New York and Mahwah, N.J.: Paulist Press.

McCormick, Richard A. 1973. Ambiguity in Moral Choice. The Pere Marquette Theology Lecture. Milwaukee: Marquette University Theology Department.

———. 1974. To Save or Let Die. *Journal of the American Medical Association* 229: 172–76. Also published in *America* 131 (July 7, 1974).

———. 1978. The Quality of Life, the Sanctity of Life. *Hastings Center Report* 8 (February 1978): 30–36.

———. 1981a. *How Brave a New World? Dilemmas in Bioethics*. Garden City, N.Y.: Doubleday.

———. 1981b. *Notes on Moral Theology, 1965 through 1980*. Washington, D.C.: University Press of America.

———. 1983. Notes on Moral Theology: 1982. *Theological Studies* 44 (March 1982): 71–122.

———. 1984a. *Health and Medicine in the Catholic Tradition: Tradition in Transition*. New York: Crossroad.

———. 1984b. Notes on Moral Theology: 1983. *Theological Studies* 45 (March 1983) 80–138.

————. 1989. *The Critical Calling: Reflections on Moral Dilemmas since Vatican II.* Washington, D.C.: Georgetown University Press.

————. 1990. Clear and Convincing Evidence: The Case of Nancy Cruzan. *Midwest Medical Ethics* 6 (fall 1990): 10–12. Also published in *Corrective Vision* (McCormick 1994).

————. 1994. *Corrective Vision: Explorations in Moral Theology.* Kansas City: Sheed and Ward.

————. 1997. A Family Member Helps a Patient Stop Breathing. In *How Shall We Die? Helping Christians Debate Assisted Suicide*, edited by Sally B. Geis and Donald E. Messer. Nashville: Abingdon.

McCormick, Richard, and André Hellegers. 1977. Legislation and the Living Will. *America* 136 (March 12, 1977): 210–13.

McCormick, Richard, and John Paris. 1983. Saving Defective Infants: Options for Life or Death. *America* (April 23, 1983): 313–17.

————. 1987. The Catholic Tradition on the Use of Nutrition and Fluids. *America* (May 2, 1987): 356–60.

McCormick, Richard A., and Robert Veatch. 1980. Preservation of Life. *Theological Studies* 41 (June 1980): 390–96.

National Conference of Catholic Bishops. 1993. Resolution on Health Care Reform. *Origins* 23: 97, 99–102.

————. 1995. *Ethical and Religious Directives for Catholic Health Care Services.* Washington, D.C.: United States Catholic Conference.

Odozor, Paulinus Ikechekwu. 1995. *Richard A. McCormick and the Renewal of Moral Theology.* Notre Dame, Ind., and London: University of Notre Dame Press.

Pius XII. 1957. The Prolongation of Life: An Address to an International Congress of Anesthesiologists. *The Pope Speaks* 4: 393–98.

Ramsey, Paul. 1970. *The Patient as Person.* New Haven, Conn., and London: Yale University Press.

Shannon, Thomas A. 2001. Killing Them Softly with Kindness: Euthanasia Legislation in the Netherlands. *America* (October 15, 2001): 16–18.

Walter, James J., and Thomas A. Shannon. 1990. *Quality of Life: The New Medical Dilemma.* New York and Mahwah, N.J.: Paulist Press.

Wildes, Kevin W. 1996. Ordinary and Extraordinary Means and the Quality of Life. *Theological Studies* 57: 500–512.

8

Contending Images of the Healer in an Era of Turnstile Medicine

WILLIAM F. MAY

The historian Martin Marty once observed that writing a book required a single, mastering idea that informed the whole. Marty himself enjoyed the inspiration of such an idea before drafting each of his books with the speed of Mozart. My writing of *The Physician's Covenant* was quite the reverse. I wrote essays in biomedical ethics across the 1970s in response to specific invitations, which led to publication in scattered journals or books. The closest piece to a programmatic essay appeared in *The Hastings Report* (December 1975) under the title, "Code, Covenant, Contract, or Philanthropy?" All the essays that eventually made their way into the book underwent a series of growth rings beyond their original planting. At length, a way of recognizing and describing a stand of trees emerged to define the whole. But I must confess I worked less like a French gardener at Versailles, imposing a formal design on a stretch of land, than like an English gardener, turning the soil a little here, pruning there, reseeding the bare spots, and hoping for some sun and rain. The result was *The Physician's Covenant: Images of the Healer in Medical Ethics*, which Westminster Press published in 1983 and brought out in a revised edition in 2000.

HISTORICAL AND CONCEPTUAL BACKGROUND

The subtitle of the book refers to several contending images for the healer. Why resort to images—such as parent, fighter, technician, contractor, covenanter, and teacher—rather than to moral principles or theories in the attempt to reflect ethically on medical practice? Most philosophers and theologians writing in medical ethics in the early 1980s were more interested in dilemmas (hard cases) than in the great overarching images that shape the convictions and the daily practice of physicians and nurses. Typically, these ethicists examined dilemmas (such as whether to tell the truth, pull the plug, or break a confidence) and then searched for moral principles that would assist moral reasoning. For example, in early editions of their magisterial work *Principles of Biomedical Ethics* (1979), Tom Beauchamp and James Childress offered a scheme similar to that found in H. D. Aiken's essay on four "Levels of Moral Conduct" (Aiken 1982). Beauchamp and Childress described an ascent from particular judgments to rules, thence to principles, and ultimately to moral theories, in exploring the way in which conscientious people go about justifying their decisions ethically. In practice, the fourth level—theorizing—tended to yield to the third level of articulating principles, since Beauchamp and Childress differed in the theories to which they subscribed (one a utilitarian, the other a duty-based theorist); but they were able to agree on four basic principles as guides for clarifying and making decisions in biomedicine. In a wider setting, Edmund Pincoffs once called this academically dominant approach "quandary ethics" (Pincoffs 1971). It supplies conscientious decision-makers, beset by vexing choices, with principles that will help clarify and sometimes resolve their quandaries.

This approach appealed particularly to ethicists at work in professional settings. The great prestige of the case method of study in law and business schools and the clinical method of training in medical and nursing schools tended to make professionals divide the moral life up into cases; and ethicists responded with elegant work on the subjects of renal dialysis, organ transplants, gene therapy, and a host of discrete but sensational problems. The cumulative result reinforced the view that ethics chiefly examines pressing quandaries, cases, problems, dilemmas, or moral binds, and seeks to resolve them by appeal to general moral principles.

This approach came to be called (and criticized as) principle-based reasoning in biomedical ethics. Beauchamp and Childress never claimed that one could rank the principles in a fixed hierarchy or apply them deductively. Moral reflection called for the further heavy labor of specifying and balancing principles in particular cases.[1] However, enthusiasts, vastly less sophisticated than Beauchamp and Childress, sometimes seemed to reify or anthropomorphize the principles. One sometimes heard talk about "Beneficence says . . . nonmaleficence counters . . . autonomy argues"; and critics weighed in with semi-envious complaints about the "Georgetown mantra": beneficence, nonmaleficence, respect for autonomy, and justice.

I was not disposed to dismiss the Beauchamp and Childress approach, even though as a Christian ethicist I recognized that "principlism," whatever its version, would tend to remove to the background not only moral theories, but also religious narratives and commitments. A respect for general principles had the distinct advantage of serving professionals who were confessionally indeterminate and philosophically diverse, and patient populations, who were religiously pluralist and secularly various. We live in what Sheldon Wolin once described as the age of the large-scale organization (Wolin 1960, ch. 10). Professionals deliver health care today largely to strangers in the setting of hospitals. Huge institutions need general policies that will help produce reliable behavior, upon which not only specialized (and therefore mutually interdependent) colleagues but also their patients can rely. One tends to expect these standards to be relatively acceptable and independent of the accidents of personal biography, philosophical conviction, and religious disposition.

However, contrary to these general tendencies in the field, I chose to explore the role images play in interpreting healers, partly because I felt I could make my own limited contribution in this area, but also for reasons more serious than the accidents of biography. Images help us understand the metaphysical grounding (and relative ranking) we assign to principles. They also deal with the question of professional identity. Case-oriented quandary ethics deals with the question, what shall I do? Should I pull the plug or not? Should I disclose treatments not covered in the patient's health care plan? But behind many dilemmas lie the deeper questions of professional identity. Who am I? Whom shall I be? Physicians and other professionals live today in the engulfing world of the marketplace and the large-scale organization; and they prepare for their professions in the boot-camp drills of the university. What am I? A mix of technician plus entrepreneur? A careerist making my way in the headwinds and crosswinds of the corporation, or something more?

THE IMAGING OF MEDICAL PRACTICE

Images, I take it, do not merely decorate. They answer the question, whom shall I be? They help us interpret ourselves, define our roles, and give us our cues for behavior. Images for illness lie behind such phrases as: he lost his health; he suffered a heart attack; the cancer riddled him. Images also interpret the healer variously as parent, fighter, technician, contractor, covenanter, or teacher.

A specific image for the healer, such as parent or fighter, is a kind of compressed story, not a specific story about an identifiable professional, but a prototypical story to which a set of particular stories bear a family resemblance, as practitioners fashion their own decisions, careers, and justifications.

In its cognitive aspect, an image also lays bare a metaphysical setting in which people live out the bible of their lives, the basic script which is theirs. The picture of the physician as parent or fighter presupposes a sense of the human condition, and the threatening powers that encircle us, that stand at the foot of the human bed. Images touch on the metaphysical; they hint at the ultimate; they lay bare the human plight and prospect.

This metaphysical horizon, in turn, provides a silhouette for one's understanding of the moral. It justifies responses that befit the hero: to succor as a parent; to fight like a mercenary; to find refuge before human misery in one's technical competence; to covenant with the stranger; or to teach patients as students whom pain disorients and uncertainty baffles.

Needless to say, patients also figure differently in these images. They define the basic character not only of the hero but also of those with whom he or she deals and the social setting in which the story plays itself out. The parent succors the child; the fighter rescues the embattled city; the technician converts the sick host into charts and lab values; the contractor deals with consumers; the teacher seeks to illumine students distracted by pain and uncertainty.

My intellectual forerunners for this line of thinking were not the giants in philosophy who shaped biomedical ethics in North America—the utilitarian John Stuart Mill or the deontologists Immanuel Kant and W. D. Ross. Instead, twenty years before publishing *The Physician's Covenant*, I wrote my dissertation on Martin Heidegger and Albert Camus, because I found spread across their works the delineation of three basic responses to death which corresponded roughly to the three traditional responses to God in the West: openness, avoidance, or resistance. The faithful approached God with awe; sinners either fought God or fled from his presence. In the modern psyche, death had replaced God as sacral power; and we have tended to respond to disease and death either: (1) with reflexive awe before its power; or (2) by waging an all-out fight against it; or (3) by falling into patterns of avoidance and denial. Inevitably, these responses have produced three different images of the physician: as parental protector of his charges from suffering; as heroic fighter who does battle against the enemy; or, less often, as companion and guide, who, in the midst of a travail, helps enlarge the soul. Those who have read *The Physician's Covenant* will recognize that I relied more heavily on the literary traces for these responses in "The Legend of the Grand

Inquisitor," "The Death of Ivan Ilych," *The Myth of Sisyphus*, *The Plague*, *Dubliners*, *Ulysses*, and *The Sun Also Rises* than on the sometimes illegible and barely translatable prose of the German philosopher.

Images not only limn the principalities and powers against which a given pattern of medical response acquires its credibility, they also help explain the relative weighting of moral principles in practice. The parental image assumes that the stricken patient needs a parental figure who will shield and comfort patients and shoulder the burden of making decisions on their behalf. Parenting tips medical practice in the direction of the moral principle of beneficence and nonmaleficence and suppresses the principles of patient autonomy. The image slides quickly into parentalism, limiting the patient's freedom and knowledge for the purposes of doing good and of protecting the patient from anguish and harm.

Not that the parental image fails to inspire virtues worth cultivating. The image emphasizes the importance of compassion and self-sacrifice, a welcome grace note in an era of marketplace medicine. Further, the image suggests that the physician, like the good parent, must engage in a limited providential activity. The word providence, *pro-video*, entails etymologically *video*, a seeing into, *pro-video*, a seeing ahead, and, finally, making provision for. Good parenting requires all three, and healing calls for them as well: a seeing into (diagnosis); a seeing ahead (prognosis); and making provision for (therapy).

But, in the face of acute suffering and the assault of disease and death, the perception of metaphysical plight takes over. Parentalism in medicine keenly experiences the absence of divine providence and substitutes a providence of its own. However, the redefined providence it offers does not open itself to the turmoil of freedom within and the pain of suffering without. Instead, to protect its charges, this substitute providence withholds knowledge, circumvents freedom, and avoids coping with death. It exercises a tight control. The patient shrinks into the physician's property, a child, incapable of knowing his or her own good.

Thus a reaction set in, in the name of the principle of respect for autonomy. But moral criticism of the parental image was not itself image-free. The word "autonomy" derives etymologically from the Greek terms *auto* (self) and *nomos* (law or norms). Autonomy refers to governance according to the self's own laws or norms. In its original usage, the word referred not to individual self-determination but to the self-governance of city-states in their resistance to imperial power. This political metaphor prized by the Greeks later shifted in meaning with the rise of classical liberal politics in the nineteenth century, which associated the self with an expansive and indeterminate liberty largely free of external constraints. In effect, modern moralists fought against the familial metaphor—the parent—with a political metaphor—self-governance. Moral argument rarely goes on at a level utterly free of image and metaphor.

We need not explore at length the dynamics by which other images reflect metaphysical perception and define the role of the healer. Suffice it to note in passing that Camus did not invent the role of the professional as fighter. Long before Camus, the military metaphor had its roots in ancient shamanic practice, as the healer fought against the negative, invasive, demonic power of disease and death. The military image resurfaced again in the modern world with the perception of viruses and bacteria that wreak havoc in the body and the use of weapons, such as modern surgery, antibiotics, and immunosuppressive drugs, with which to fight against destructive power.

Eventually, modern medicine tended to interpret itself not only through the prism of war but through the medium of its twentieth-century practice, that is, unlimited war. The patient only too often resembled the Vietnam village utterly flattened in the course of liberating it.

Once again, a reaction set in. Patients and families, and eventually some practitioners, wanted to set limits to the battle against death. The federal government encouraged the development of hospital policies on end of life care. Funding agencies also weighed in. The government instituted budgetary constraints on the war through the device of diagnostically related groups; and insurance companies and prepayment providers curtailed rapidly growing outlays to finance the battle.

Thus the parental and military images increasingly yielded in the 1990s to a less heroic, composite portrait of the physician as a *technician* plus *contractor*. Physicians acquire through a long period of arduous training their technical skills, which they are then free to sell as advantageously as they can through a fee-for-service or prepayment system. A commercial contract largely defines the range and limits of their services.

The first aspect of the composite image—the ideal of excellence in technical performance—deserves more positive appreciation than it usually receives from ethicists today. It dates all the way back to the Hippocratic emphasis on *philotechnia*, the love of the art; and it carries forward into latter-day criteria for admission to medical school, the training that prevails there, the placement of graduates in residencies, and eventual job references. All these hurdles and pressure points combine to emphasize the preeminent place of technical performance in the formation and career of the professional.

The ideal of technical skill performs valuable psychological, moral, and aesthetic functions, particularly for practitioners who must traffic daily with human sorrow and death. Under trying conditions, the ideal of technical competence helps psychologically to free the physician and nurse from the destructive consequences of too much involvement. It seems prudent to offer whatever help one can through finely honed technical services and let one's skill also provide the healer with a leaden shield against a field of radioactive emotions.

The ideal also makes its moral demands upon the professional. It requires a long period of education and training in which gratification must be delayed; and it continues to demand that the full-fledged professional subordinate the ego, its likes and its dislikes, to the technical question of how to do a thing and do it well. The technical ideal also gratifies aesthetically. It encourages a proficiency that is quietly eloquent. It conjoins the good with the beautiful. Wasted words and motion fall away; all else is subordinated to the demand on one's skill.

The second aspect of the composite image—the physician solely as the seller of his or her technical skills—fits into the contours of the current, high-tech health care system but with some disadvantageous consequences for professional identity. Under the terms of marketplace competition today, medical practice tends to be rapid-fire, illegible, specialized, and thus often disaggregated. Driven by money, the health care system also denies access to too many and has proved too imbalanced and lopsided in the services it does offer. I will explore some of these negative features of current practice with a view to their impacts on the cluster of images at the core of *The Physician's Covenant*: the healer as the practitioner of an art, not just the retailer of an applied science; the healer as teacher of his or her patients, not just the dispenser of technical services; and the healer as receiving his or her ultimate identity from an exchange of giving and receiving that transcends the cash nexus of buying and selling.

THE CONTEMPORARY SCENE

We live in an age of turnstile medicine. Whether under a fee-for-service or a prepayment system, the survival game in medicine today demands figuring out how to move people through a system fast. Under a fee-for-service system, the more rapidly providers can perform billable services, the more money the hospital and the practitioner make. Under a prepayment system, the more patients the provider can handle without having to deliver time- and equipment-expensive services, the more money the organization makes. In either case, the speed with which the turnstile clicks governs the balance sheet. "Productivity" is the buzzword in the workplace. The doctor's average contact time with patients has dropped from twenty-seven minutes to sixteen minutes and less, sometimes much less. The technique of moving people rapidly through a system has become an art. Walt Disney is its twentieth-century master. Disney's theme parks enclose an expensive piece of finite space that imposes chronic, core costs. The firm makes money by moving people through the system efficiently and rapidly. (I used to belong to a golf club that learned its lesson from Disney. The corporation that owns the club has kept trees to a minimum. Why? Trees block shots; trees also shed leaves, a habit that makes balls hard to find; thus trees slow up the game. Increase the trees and golf scores will be higher, players less happy, the playing time longer, and the course unable to support as many members and thus yield as large a profit to owners.) After I offered some of these remarks in the course of grand rounds at a distinguished tertiary care hospital, my hosts reported that the hospital had invited in as consultants a few weeks earlier two experts from the Disney Corporation. Learning how to hustle people happily through a system loomed large in the hospital's effort to survive.

The economic pressure to keep everything up to speed affects two images of medicine explored in *The Physician's Covenant*. First, turnstile medicine emphasizes healing as an applied science rather than sustains it as an art. We can argue the claim that medicine is an art either weakly and provisionally or strongly and intrinsically. In its weaker form, we describe medicine as an art only temporarily in the sense that we have not yet perfected it as a science. In its stronger form, we claim that healing is an art not merely provisionally but intrinsically. It must remain an art. A scientist traffics in universals and therefore must abstract from the particular. To achieve its generalization, a scientific hypothesis must abstract from the complexity of the universe; it selects for description a particular set of recurrent phenomena, isolated from all the variables in which they might be embedded, and seeks to arrive at a generalization that covers the phenomena under scrutiny. Science reduces water to the abstract formula of H_2O. The poet Yeats complained, I like a little seaweed in my definition of water. Artists wrestle with the concrete; they leave in some variables. They offer not universals but a concrete universe—Lear's universe, Antigone's world, and Michelangelo's Pieta.

We can define healing as an art because the individual patient whom the healer serves does not merely illustrate a general scientific principle into which the patient entirely disappears. Each patient is a full-bodied person with her own history and universe, seaweed and all. Her diabetes may, more or less, illustrate a generalization about the particular disease. But we cannot tidily abstract the host from the disease or the disease from the host.

Diagnosing and treating the disease and helping the ill person face her disease require knowing the patient, her habits, her world, her pressures and strains.[2] These complex undertakings surely draw on science, but the physician must artfully marshal the generalizations of science to heal the person rather than merely treat the disease. The healer cannot prescind from the universe that accompanies the patient in order to handle a detail that fits and confirms an abstract rule.

Institutional pressures today favor interpreting medicine solely as a retailable, applied science. The reduction of medicine to an applied science fits conveniently into the current corporatization of health care. If doctoring merely applies science or technical expertise, then one can diagnose, treat, and heal at a distance, the very considerable distance of an 800 number, for instance, with a case manager at the other end of the phone and with a recipe book in hand. The doctor becomes retailer and dispenser of interventions authorized elsewhere.

But, as a psychiatrist remarked to me, every thoughtful psychiatrist knows that the better you get to know a patient, the more difficult it is to classify him under one of the diseases listed in the DSM IV.[3] The patient does not conveniently vanish into the scientist's law. The doctor uses science, but healing also requires practical wisdom in bringing science artfully to bear in order to restore harmony to the patient's universe. Such healing is the end purpose of doctoring, and it takes time.

Turnstile medicine also tends to neglect the teaching responsibilities of physicians and nurses, a responsibility highlighted in *The Physician's Covenant* in the chapter on the "Physician as Teacher." Rapid-fire treatment organizes doctors and others as dispensers of technical services rather than teachers of their patients. Teaching is important not only in securing compliance with acute care interventions but in helping patients face the great alterations in life that often accompany rehabilitative, long-term, and terminal care, and the reconstruction of habits necessitated by preventive medicine. But teaching takes time. It is slow boring through hard wood.

Illegible

Medical services today are increasingly illegible. They lack transparency. We live in what we take pride in calling an Information Age, yet an age in which both workers producing goods and services and the recipients of the goods and services often do not have the means of understanding them or their functions. In *The Corrosion of Character*, Richard Sennett contrasts the relatively knowledgeable traditional baker, preparing his breads, with the clueless modern employee of a large bakery (Sennett 1998). The latter serves preset machines but without knowledge as to how bread is made or how the machines work. He merely tends to some aspect of a largely opaque operation. More darkly, the Enron Corporation has shown how corporations can exploit illegibility—in Enron's case, manipulating energy markets and concocting off-shore partnerships designed to obscure losses and gains and inflate profits. The practice rendered Enron's corporate operations utterly opaque, not only to unsophisticated investors in the world at large but to workers within its own glass walls, and, if reports and claims are correct, inaccessible even to market analysts and investment experts. In the Enron case, mendacity and rapacity exploited opacity, but opacity alone is unsettling enough. Ordinary folk can be especially rattled, living in a world that is largely unreadable and then suddenly faced with a medical crisis that poses vexing and competing choices for them in the treatment of prostate cancer, breast cancer, or a low-birth-weight infant in a neonatal intensive care unit. The assault of disease confounds them and professionals buzz about them, drawing upon a very complex and esoteric body of knowledge that reminds patients and their families only of their inadequate preparation for rapid sight reading.

Thus the anxieties of patients and families heighten, and distrust shadows their relationship even to well-intentioned practitioners. Cumulatively, the rapidity with which professionals render services and the illegibility of what they offer intensify the need for physicians who are not simply technicians but wise teachers of their patients and their families. Moreover, to engage in teaching that builds trust, physicians must not only be masters of a body of knowledge but respect their patients sufficiently to read them attentively. Otherwise, an opaque body of knowledge collides with a patient who is opaque, his needs unread except for what shows up in lab values.

Services Highly Specialized but Often Disaggregated

Until recently in the United States, 70 percent of physicians were specialists and only 30 percent were generalists. In other industrial nations, the ratios were the reverse or closer to 50-50 in the distribution of specialists to generalists. Highly specialized medical practice in the United States has performed brilliantly in producing particular outcomes, but services sometimes seem to disaggregate. We cannot reasonably expect that each and every specialist will know the patient's habits, world, pressures, and strains. Specialists operate within the boundaries of their technical competence where they can contribute limitedly but importantly to the total array of scientific information that assists effective treatment. But in the era of fragmented diagnostic services and often competing treatment options, directorial responsibility must be located somewhere. Otherwise, the patient can find himself cut adrift, acting somewhat anxiously as his own primary care physician and making fateful choices without the steadying presence of a healer.

Thus, in the first edition of *The Physician's Covenant*, I recognized the need to write about covenanted institutions, not simply covenanted individual practitioners. As a practical matter, the patient especially needs a coherent health care team. However, the physician who serves as captain of the team has received an education that chiefly hones his or her technical skills; it does not prepare the physician thoroughly for directorial responsibilities. It is as if the first violinist of an orchestra (the most technically demanding role) also had to serve as conductor of the orchestra, without much preparation for the latter post. Only too often the strategist, preoccupied with his or her own work as a specialist, lets the comprehensive strategy lie undeveloped. Absent directorial intelligence, an unauthorized nurse, or the patient herself, or a family member finds herself in the lonely position of conductor of the orchestra, without quite knowing the score and lacking any sense of continuity from one musical phrase or phase to the next—an oboe here, a clarinet there, a violin to the left, a second bass fiddle to the right. It's lonely and isolating up there at the podium.

Physicians adequately prepared for leadership can help provide continuity and coherence in health care. Thoughtful policy guidelines and correct institutional procedures can also help. But fidelity to the patient and the patient's plight also requires a brace of personal virtues, apart from which high-strung professionals will find it difficult to make a health care team or a hospital work. At a minimum, these virtues include a measure of charity and good faith in dealing with an irritating colleague; a good dose of caution in heeding a friend who only too quickly approves what we say or do; some humility before the powers we wield for good or for ill; the discipline to seek wisdom rather than showing off by

scoring points; sufficient integrity not to pretend to more certainty than
we have; and enough bravery to act when we must, even in the midst
of uncertainty.

THE PROFESSIONAL AND SOCIETAL COVENANT

What I have said about healing as an art and about the teaching responsibilities of practitioners and about the kinds of virtues they require delves
into matters that cannot be fully detailed in a commercial contract. I
believe it finally rests on a sense of professional identity derived from an
exchange of giving and receiving that exceeds the cash nexus of buying
and selling. I have called this further obligation and this requisite seasoning
of the virtues *covenantal fidelity*.

The Hippocratic tradition limitedly adumbrated this deeper level of
obligation when it described the young physician as receiving a huge gift
from his teacher who initiates him into the art of healing—a gift beyond
repayment which elicits from the young physician a covenantal loyalty. I
am not proposing that physicians ride down the moonbeams of nostalgia
and embrace the details of the Hippocratic oath. But I do want to call
attention to the fundamental insight of a covenantal tradition, which
appears even more forcibly and comprehensively in the biblical traditions
of the Near East and West and carries forward in the work of the twentieth-
century theologians Karl Barth and Paul Ramsey and the novelist William
Faulkner. This tradition affirms that beneath the commercial and contractual world of buying and selling that characterizes so much of human
life—the disposition of land and the sale and purchase of goods and
services—a much deeper tie of giving and receiving binds human beings to
one another and to the land they till and the air they breathe. Professionals
function at both levels, contractual and covenantal. They earn their living
by their work and it would be a species of angelism to deny this fact. But
they also benefit, more richly than most, from the bestowals of life and
learning and talent and sociality and nurture for which they are answerable,
and answerable to a degree far beyond the commercial transactions into
which they enter and the occasional works of charity with which they
airbrush their lives and careers.

Specifically, professionals work very hard to acquire their education
and their identity. But the knowledge-based power which they wield does
not spring independently from their foreheads. It is not self-derived. No
professional can go through a modern university and plausibly pretend
to be a self-made man or woman. A huge company of men and women,

humble and mighty, contributes to the shaping of professionals as they zigzag their way through childhood, college, and professional schools. One cannot, of course, fully appreciate this covenantal indebtedness of human beings by toting up the varying sacrifices and investments of others from which they benefit. The sense that one inexhaustibly receives presupposes an infinite inexhaustible source rather than a finite sum of discrete gifts received from others. Still, the secondary gifts in the human order of giving and receiving, in which professionals participate, can strengthen their sense of covenantal obligation.

A nineteenth-century visitor to this country, Alexis de Tocqueville, pointed to a larger societal covenant that characterizes American life at its best: "A covenant exists . . . between all the citizens of a democracy when they all feel themselves subject to the same weakness and the same dangers; their interests as well as compassion makes it a rule with them to lend one another assistance when required."

Such a covenantal sense of responsibility hardly supplies specific directives for the design of a health care system, in the sense, for example, of insisting on a single-payer system, as opposed to some other type, for funding and distributing health care. However, it supplies directions, if not directives, that require us to respect three basic features of health care: it is a fundamental good; it is not the only fundamental good; and it is a public good.

Because health care is a fundamental good (not an optional commodity like a Walkman, a tie, or a scarf), it ought to offer universal access and a comprehensive range of services. The covenant cannot exclude.

Because health care is not the only fundamental good and it competes with other fundamental and higher goods, it must be efficient and cost-effective. Efficiency and cost-effectiveness are not simply economic but moral considerations. The covenant ought not waste.

Because it is a public good, reflecting a huge public investment, a health care system must increase the practitioner's sense of responsibility for the skill he or she exercises as a calling, not simply as a career, and the patient's sense of responsibility for collaborative self-care. The covenant engages each in a calling.

Finally, any such covenanted system must respect its limits. No matter how ingeniously devised, it cannot gratify all wants, tamp down all worries, or remove the mark of mortality from our frame. It is a cliché to say that physicians ought not to play God. Neither should a health care system indulge an aspiration to immortality.

NOTES

1. For an able defense of their principle-based approach to biomedical ethics, see Childress 1997.

2. Eric Cassell writes: "Disease . . . is something an organ has; illness is something a man has" (Cassell 1979, 48).

3. The *Diagnostic and Statistical Manual of Mental Disorders*, fourth edition (1994), which describes and classifies mental illnesses and emotional disorders.

REFERENCES

Aiken, H. D., ed. 1982. *Reason and Conduct: New Bearings in Moral Philosophy.* Westport, Conn.: Greenwood Press.

Beauchamp, Tom L., and James F. Childress. 1979. *Principles of Biomedical Ethics.* New York: Oxford University Press.

Cassell, Eric. 1979. *The Healer's Art.* New York: Penguin Books.

Childress, James F. 1997. The Normative Principles of Medical Ethics. In *Medical Ethics*, edited by R. M. Veatch. Sudbury, Mass.: Jones and Bartlett Publishers.

May, William F. 1975. Code, Covenant, Contract, or Philanthropy? *The Hastings Center Report* 5 (December 1975): 29–38.

———. 1983. *The Physician's Covenant.* Philadelphia: Westminster Press.

———. 2000. *The Physician's Covenant.* Revised edition. Philadelphia: Westminster Press.

Pincoffs, Edmund. 1971. Quandary Ethics. *Mind* 80: 552–71.

Sennett, Richard. 1998. *The Corrosion of Character: Personal Development in the New Capitalism.* New York: W. W. Norton and Co.

Wolin, Sheldon. 1960. *Politics and Vision.* Boston: Little, Brown and Co.

PART THREE

Boundaries and Issues of Inclusion in Bioethics

Shaping and Mirroring the Field: The *Encyclopedia of Bioethics*

WARREN T. REICH

Published and unpublished comments on the role and significance of the *Encyclopedia of Bioethics* (referred to hereafter as *EB*) that have been made over the past twenty-five years by numerous leaders in the field have established the following summary description: that the first edition of the *EB* (Reich 1978) played a major role in establishing the field of bioethics, formulated the most widely accepted definition of bioethics, defined the scope of the field, provided the first organization of knowledge for this field, and articulated standards for bioethics scholarship.

In the late 1980s, when I was trying to determine whether and how to perpetuate the *EB*—through a consultation process that led to the creation of the second edition (Reich 1995)—Daniel Callahan commented that in addition to being a constantly used reference tool, the *EB* "has served as a very important central document, providing unity, coherence, and direction for the field that one might never get from simply consulting the assorted books and articles that make up most fields."[1] Callahan's comment evokes the theme I would like to pursue in this essay on the past and future of the *EB*: the enormous responsibility that has been placed on the shoulders of some bioethicists to take attentive care of the central unifying documents of the field, and how that responsibility over time creates a sense of responsibility of caring for the field of bioethics itself.

How to carry out that responsibility depends on how one specifies what the *EB* should accomplish. I regard the first edition of the *EB* as having had the function of *shaping* the field, while the second edition began the process of *mirroring* the field while continuing the function of shaping it. I believe it is essential that neither pole of these contrasting functions ever be abandoned. As time goes on, there will be more and more pressure to see to it that the *EB* simply *mirrors* and accurately summarizes ongoing developments in the field; but responsibility for the field requires that the *EB* continue to creatively *shape* the field as well.

INSPIRATION FOR THE *ENCYCLOPEDIA* OF *BIOETHICS*

I initiated the *EB* out of desperation. I had to have some project to pursue at the then–brand-new Kennedy Institute of Ethics, whose founding director, André Hellegers, had a vision of simply recruiting some bright people and facilitating their attempts to do whatever they thought worthwhile. But there was no model for me to follow, for in mid-1971 no one had blazed that trail before me.

In retrospect, I think a major factor that drew me in the direction of developing the idea for an encyclopedia was the fact that when I arrived at the Kennedy Institute I had lost a sense of my broader intellectual agenda. A few years earlier, as a faculty member at The Catholic University of America, I had taken part in closing down the university in protest against one violation of academic freedom, and then having to defend my own academic freedom and that of nineteen professor-colleagues in a year-long inquiry into the acceptability of having publicly articulated, on the grounds of our own theological discipline, the practical limits of the authoritative force of a monumentally important papal pronouncement against birth control. Thus, when I came to Georgetown as a "dissenter," I felt radically disconnected from my past academic pursuits and had no clear vision of my professional or intellectual future. Furthermore, after the 1960s I felt that I, together with countless others throughout the world, was experiencing the decisive end of one cultural, moral, and social era and the beginning of another, the contours of which were not yet defined. Thirty-one years later, I see that my serendipitous situation of being suspended between cultures in 1971 was precisely the requisite spiritual and intellectual condition for the task of trying to absorb and articulate the contours, meanings, and normative issues of a new social, intellectual, and political reality that was rapidly taking shape before our very eyes, the future of which we did not know.

Another reason for conceptualizing and undertaking this work was my own curiosity. In mid-1971, as André Hellegers, LeRoy Walters, and I were launching the Kennedy Institute, I felt a rush of enormous curiosity not so much regarding a specific bioethical topic as the totality of what was appearing on the intellectual horizon. I recall stepping back and asking over and over again: What is really going on here? Why are these problems in science and medicine not simply appearing one by one, seeking solutions, but coalescing socially, culturally, politically, and intellectually around this new concept bioethics? I wondered: Where will people turn for intellectual guidance for new moral questions like the Jewish Chronic Disease hospital case of deceptive human experimentation, the decision to abandon the care of certain handicapped infants, the prospect of some day creating babies in a test tube, and the thousands of issues affecting life, death, and health that one could perceive just beyond the horizon of contemporaneous controversy? I decided to respond to my own question by assembling and organizing the knowledge that would be needed for the bioethics that seemed to be appearing. My goal was to reach far into all the corners of the worlds of the life sciences and ethics to expose all the moral issues for careful ethical scrutiny, and to provide the philosophical, religious, and social underpinnings for the major discussions. It is hard to convey today how terribly naive that decision was, yet I eventually came to respect naiveté as an indispensable tool for accomplishing a complex project in uncharted territory. Later I came to realize that in this I was not unique; most often, unprecedented syntheses of knowledge in specialized fields of learning are developed by scholars within the field who have never before undertaken such a work.

IDEAS THAT INFLUENCED
THE ORIGINS OF THE *EB* PROJECT

The following ideas and traditions from my own background were influential factors in the creation of the *EB*: (1) Training in the systematic and comprehensive methods of Catholic medical ethics and moral theology, perhaps the most extensively developed, systematic approach to those areas of learning at that time. (2) An allegiance to the indispensable role of rigorous rational inquiry in ethics, religion, and science. (3) A commitment to the link between the ethical and the pastoral, i.e., the conviction that there should be no intellectual or disciplinary wall between the rational construction of ethics and the morality of the care of the whole person in the troubled reality of her life. (4) A growing awareness of the inherently pluralistic character of ethical inquiry, as a result of the profound intellectual impact of the secularization and ecumenical movements of the 1960s. (5) An antiminimalist commitment shaped in the 1950s and 1960s by the dramatic watershed turn from legalistic, rule-based ethics in theology to a richer set of ideals (such as love) on the one hand and a more contextual appreciation of moral decision making on the other. (6) The conviction that ethics must be prepared to be countercultural, ready to challenge the moral priorities of the powerful institutions—the state, the church, the professions, and the military—a conviction shaped by the prophetic religious tradition and reinforced by the influence of Marxist ethics in the 1960s. (7) A fierce personal commitment to freedom of expression and to hearing all voices, if necessary by inviting hitherto unheard voices to the dialogue. Because of my own experience, I was determined that no religious, philosophical, or ideological bias would be allowed to inflate or exclude any contribution to this first reference work in the field. For those times, a commitment of that sort was crucially important if the resulting encyclopedia, prepared at a Catholic university by a scholar trained principally in Catholic moral theology, together with a group of editors the majority of whom had training in religious ethics, was to be credible.

Those governing ideas and commitments had the effect of both respecting and questioning received traditions and ideas, ferreting out for discussion problems that had previously been somewhat avoided, and reaching for neglected and new approaches to ethical reflection. My colleagues and I, working from a revisionist, expansive ethical outlook, knew that we were establishing a secular bioethics in which both philosophical and religious ethics would participate, along with the other relevant scientific and humanistic disciplines. These ideas and commitments were reinforced by the Kennedy Foundation's motivation to create a link between values and science and the dedication to bringing the biomedical sciences and normative disciplines into dialogue on the part of André Hellegers, the Kennedy Institute's founding director.

CONCEPTUALIZING THE FUNCTION OF THE *ENCYCLOPEDIA*

The most basic principle to which I often reverted in establishing the objectives and standards for developing the *EB* was embodied, for me, in the word encyclopedia, which is composed of two Greek words, *enkuklios paideia*. I took the word *paideia*, which means the formal educational training of youth in the arts and sciences, as an indicator of the responsibility to create a comprehensive assemblage of all the knowledge, both general and specific, that would be needed for bioethics as a field of learning and an area of responsible action at individual, social, political, and professional levels. This principle of comprehensive coverage drove me to fear that we might overlook some problems of professionals, scientists, environmentalists, parents, or anyone concerned about ethics and the life sciences conceived in the broadest possible terms. I interpreted the term *enkuklios* (encyclo-), or cyclic, to signify a rather simple notion of "circle of learning," in the sense that we must organize the information in such a way that an uninitiated person could move easily from one set of information to another, travelling, so to speak, in a circle from article to article in search of more and more complete knowledge of a given topic, with the size of the circle to be determined by the interests of the searcher. For example, the search for a practical issue like genetic research could lead the reader to the scientific underpinnings, to the religious and philosophical principles involved, to the legal and social standards, to related practical issues of clinic or environment, and then back to the problem area with which one started, thus completing the circle.

After all the textual pieces of the *EB* had been assembled, the experience of finalizing the architectonics of bioethics—symbolized by the cross-referencing, blind (*See*) entries, and indexing, and schematized in the "Systematic Classification of Articles" at the end of the work—provided an enormous satisfaction. Too bad, I often thought, that the architectonics manifesting the *enkuklios* of this work remained virtually invisible to many readers and practically all reviewers. For some of us, though, it meant that finally the field of bioethics itself had wholeness and structure and an integrity to be tended to, even if this integrity had the limitations of this one architectonic scheme.

PREPARATION AND RECEPTION OF THE ENCYCLOPEDIA

The first, pioneering edition of the *EB* was the result of a collaborative effort by a group of eight outstanding associate editors who were charged with the responsibility of planning and reviewing the various topical areas of bioethics. They were: K. Danner Clouser, H. Tristram Engelhardt, Jr., John C. Fletcher, Stanley Hauerwas, Albert R. Jonsen, Robert Neville, Robert M. Veatch, and LeRoy Walters. I was greatly relieved when they agreed to collaborate; each one of them was my first choice for a specific area of expertise. It was a remarkably young group of scholars. For example, Tristram Engelhardt, just one year out of his Ph.D. studies, had written only one paper on a philosophical topic (personhood) related to bioethics. LeRoy Walters had come to Georgetown straight out of graduate school; but prior to starting work on the *EB* he had developed the first bibliography of bioethics and started the Bioethics Library. (The library, together with other Walters-directed projects including the multivolume *Bibliography of Bioethics* and the Bioethics Information Retrieval System, would become extraordinarily valuable in-house tools for developing the *EB*.) The work would never have succeeded without the extensive expertise, intellectual commitment, and generous collaborative spirit of this exceptional team of scholars. The project owed an enormous debt to managing editor Sandra M. Hass, and to James J. Doyle, assistant editor, not only for their superb and loyal work, but also because each of them constantly urged us and cheered us on to the high standards that eventually characterized the work.

Many of the first-edition articles were the first ever published on their topic, a situation most unusual for an encyclopedia yet necessary for one whose task it was to codify a new field of learning. For example, at a time when the notion of care was almost totally undeveloped—only one significant work on the philosophy of care existed at the time (Mayeroff 1971)—Stanley Hauerwas prepared a classic, original article on what care could mean in a health context. Arthur L. Basham prepared an unprecedented comprehensive article on bioethics in Hinduism; and Albert Jonsen did the principal planning for a series of twenty-nine articles that constituted the first comprehensive compilation of the history of medical ethics. The goal of our editorial team was to prepare a work that would be characterized by the comprehensiveness and accuracy that speak to the specialist, coupled with the accessibility of style required for the broad dissemination of knowledge.

The most important reviews of the first edition were thorough ones by established scholars who reviewed the work positively but also offered the most important challenges and criticisms. For example, the most thorough review of all, by David Schenck, Glenn Graber, and Charles Reynolds, assessed the *EB* as "accurate" and "accessible"; "outstanding" in terms of clarity, scope, and accessibility; and "the most significant contribution to solid foundations for the field that has yet appeared." However, opting to review the young and expanding field of bioethics itself "as mirrored . . . quite faithfully . . . in this massive text," they criticized the tendency they found in the *EB*, evidenced most clearly in Clouser's article on "Bioethics," of conceiving bioethics as applying the known principles of what Clouser called "the same old ethics" that was shaped by what the reviewers called "the unreconstructed canonical works of Kant and Mill" to a particular realm of concerns. They also faulted the *EB*'s corresponding failure to foresee and integrate in itself the impact of the life sciences on values and ethics and "the rootedness of values and principles in specific social contexts, e.g., the professional practice of medicine." They noted that the *EB* included information from medical sociology and anthropology but without synthesizing these resources in ethical analyses (Schenck, Graber, and Reynolds 1981). Although I believe the first edition of the *EB* advanced the integration of knowledge beyond what these reviewers perceived in the field generally, their comments on the fundamental neglect of interdisciplinary synthesis in bioethics, which presaged extensive criticisms of the field that have been made in the intervening years, can and should continue to serve as a standard for the dynamic intellectual creativity that should be occurring among all the disciplines represented within the field of bioethics—a creativity that should be both reported and advanced by the *EB*.

The second edition of the *EB* represented an enormous advancement over the first edition. Incorrectly called a revised edition (it was an almost totally new and considerably expanded edition), it was at least twice as difficult to accomplish as the first edition had been, partly because it required matching and exceeding the reception the first edition had been accorded, and partly because the field of bioethics had changed so extensively in the years between publication of the first edition (1978) and commencement of the second edition (1990). The dramatic changes in the field of bioethics were due not only to scientific and medical "advances" and an almost total change in relevant legal components, but because ethics itself had evolved so much in the intervening years.

To establish whether and how to keep the *EB* alive and useful, I carried out a two-year research and consultation process in the late 1980s, funded by the National Endowment for the Humanities. I then drew up a plan for the whole work, selected the smartest possible Area Editors, and asked them to draw up detailed plans for each section, which I integrated and coordinated into a unified work. The Area Editors were Dan Beauchamp, Arthur Caplan, Christine Cassell, James F. Childress, Allen R. Dyer, John C. Fletcher, Stanley Hauerwas, Albert R. Jonsen, Patricia King, Loretta Kopelman, Ruth Purtilo, Holmes Rolston III, Robert M. Veatch, and Donald P. Warwick.[2] Stephen Post, who filled a crucially important new position called "associate editor," worked very effectively with the editor-in-chief; and Mary Evans, the extremely resourceful coordinating editor, was, along with Post, my constant dialogue partner on methods and quality. Mary Solberg, a highly skilled editor and scholar, was the magical managing editor in New York.

Whereas the 1978 edition contained 315 articles by 285 contributors in four volumes, the 1995 edition was expanded to 464 articles by 437 contributors in five volumes. Only a few classic first-edition articles—by intellectual luminaries such as Talcott Parson, Pedro Laín Entralgo, Jay Katz, and Joseph Kitagawa—were carried over to the second edition. I have no doubt that the second edition established the *EB* on a new and higher plane and signaled a much stronger standing for the field. The published reviews were quite favorable and some were very instructive for the future of the *EB* and for the field as a whole (Christie, Davis, and Twiss 1996; Koczwara and Madigan 1997).

THE FUTURE OF THE ENCYCLOPEDIA

What should be the future of the *EB*? I believe it should not be taken for granted that the *EB* should be perpetuated. Most books and even many reference tools have a limited life; and since bioethics may turn to other "central documents" as its favored reference tools, depending on need and the desired medium, the case needs to be made over and over again whether and how the *EB* should be maintained. For the present, from the consulting I have done and the impression I have from conversations in various parts of the world, I believe the *EB* is still a viable and valued tool worthy of revision. Hardbound books seem still to be a staple source of information; and the various sources available on the Internet do not offer comprehensive and high-quality information. I have striven unsuccessfully for over fifteen years to persuade the publisher (Macmillan Reference, now part of the Gale Group) to put the *EB* online, with arrangements made to update sections of the work every six months or so. In the meantime, the *EB* should, for the foreseeable future, be kept alive through preparation of further editions; and in fact, the third edition is now in its early stages of preparation.[3]

What sort of an *EB* future scholars will create depends on how they regard its legacy; and in this regard the comments of Peter Steinfels are instructive. Recalling that Denis Diderot wrote in 1755 that the task of an encyclopedia was nothing less than "to change the general way of thinking," Steinfels commented that the *EB* was a "major event," promising "to carry out Diderot's lofty assignment," because it compressed into four volumes the way that bioethics itself had been "changing our way of thinking" by "urging the cause of serious reflection and discussion generally" (Steinfels 1979, 40–41). Was that "lofty assignment" only a one-time function of the past? Does the *EB* still have the function of continuing to change the general way of thinking, both within the field of bioethics and in other areas of public and applied ethics that it spawned? Scholars who undertake to keep this instrument alive would do well to address this challenging question.

Planning for the future of the *EB* must take into account the number, foci, and quality of the great number of reference works covering all or parts of bioethics that have appeared in the past thirty years. My own survey of this extensive literature leads me to single out three leading works published in three foreign languages that are instructive for planning not only the international dimensions but also the totality of the *EB*. They are the *Lexikon der Bioethik* by Wilhelm Korff and colleagues (Korff 1998), which is especially instructive regarding its expansive range of topics; the *Nouvelle encyclopedie de bioethique* by Gilbert Hottois and colleagues (Hottois 2001), especially praiseworthy for its organization around medicine, the environment, and biotechnology; and *Ethiek & Recht in de Gezondheidszorg* (ten Have 1992), which is restricted to health care ethics and proves that a systematic arrangement can sometimes give shape to a more useful reference tool than an alphabetical arrangement. Although it may be impossible to prepare a fully international encyclopedia of bioethics due to differing moral beliefs, ethics, and laws in the various parts of the world—which are the reasons why the 1995 edition of the *EB* was not able to become a fully satisfactory international tool—I believe there is still need for a bioethics reference work, preferably published in English, that continues to approximate as international and intercultural a scope as possible; and I think that tool remains the *EB*, until it is replaced by a more effective international reference instrument.

The remainder of my comments will be in the form of my recommendations as to what topics (placed within quotation marks) are of great significance for the field of bioethics and consequently should be addressed in the next edition of the *EB*.[4] I will cite random sources published, for the most part, since 1995 (publication date of the second edition), not all of equal value, that are evidence of the sorts of topics that should be addressed and why.

There are many topics that unproblematically require inclusion or serious renovation in the third edition—topics that any competent group of editors would in fact want to include in the bioethical canon. They include practical problems such as "cloning," "stem-cell research," "genome mapping and sequencing," and "genetic engineering," with targeted attention to extraordinarily important issues such as those raised by "gene therapy" and "gene-altered food." The catastrophic events of September 11, 2001, necessitate an entry on "bioterrorism" and sharpen our attention to the neglected but growing area of "public health ethics" (Beauchamp and Steinbock 1999) and "public health law" (Gostin 2000). Additional newer topics that deserve inclusion are "biodiversity," "infertility," "palliative care," "preventive medicine," "parental consent/notification," and several world religions: "Shintoism" (previously discussed in the article on the history of medical ethics in Japan through the nineteenth century) and "Zoroastrianism." "Poverty" (social, economic, political, philosophical, religious, and ethical considerations, nationally and globally) is an extraordinarily important, yet neglected topic. Widespread international consternation over "health-care delivery" and "managed care" require revision of the relevant entries. The entry on the "professional-patient relationship" should reflect a more creative crossing of professional boundaries—for example, by applying the developmental model of nursing skills to medicine and other professions (Benner 1984). Finally, I have no worry at all that any group of future editors would commission excellent entries on "bioethics" and "ethics" that will report on and offer creative syntheses of the debates regarding the role of principles, virtues, care, etc., in bioethical discourse.

A CRITERION FOR SALIENCE IN THE *EB*: THE ROLE OF EXPERIENCE

On the other hand, I do worry about how bioethical attention is directed to the field as a whole. While encyclopedists must refrain from shaping the reference work according to their own preferred approaches to the field, I am convinced that a commitment to the central role played by experience in ethics—the interpretation and understanding of moral experience and the general and specific responses to it—is an extraordinarily useful starting-point for providing an answer to the formal question: What sorts of issues and responses should be included in an encyclopedia that is regarded as the central document of the field and that needs to be retooled to meet the needs of bioethics in the present and in the era that is now commencing?

Children provide an appropriate starting point for a consideration of why certain topics are systematically neglected in bioethics. When I surveyed the bioethics literature for a recent five-year period to see what bioethicists are saying about children, I discovered, not surprisingly, that over 90 percent of the literature dealt with consent in and for children. Although some noteworthy attempts have been made to deal with the neglect of children in bioethics (Mahowald 1993; Murray 1996; Michel 1999), the field of bioethics as a whole has neglected most problems related to children, including the sexual, physical, and psychological abuse of children all over the world and the neglect of the care of children, both of which lead to injury, disease, and threats to the lives of children.

I believe the underlying reason for this neglect is that bioethics has largely been held captive by a highly restrictive conceptual framework that effectively excludes a consideration of the experiences of children and of those who relate to children. Bioethics is strongly shaped, in both its philosophical and scientific roots, by a scientifically constructed knowledge which is not compatible with the situated logic and rationality that inform our ways of understanding the socioculturally constituted meaning of the experiences of children and other vulnerable populations (Kirkengen 2001). This explanation, in turn, is instructive regarding bioethical selectivity and exclusion in many other areas of moral experience. However one may view the problem of topical selectivity and the intellectual and educational organization of our field, those who are responsible for a document that purports to present bioethics comprehensively must be circumspect and at times intellectually countercultural to their own field in order to show fair and creative attention to the full range of issues and populations. The sort of attentiveness that shapes the field of bioethics and its various texts hinges on the deeper question, whether ordinary human experience—primary experience, as distinct from experience that has already been intellectually processed and systematized—has a place in ethics, philosophy, and theology.

This question signals the turning point at which bioethics currently finds itself, for we have been witnessing over the past twenty years or so a great intellectual revolution surrounding the role of experience, evidenced in a special way in bioethics. The term *revolution* is a sober description, considering the history of the debate. The Western philosophical tradition, from its very beginnings, has been an intellectual force for downgrading ordinary, everyday experience (Reed 1996, 13). "For Plato the abstract idea of a thing . . . is what is truly real; our world here is but a shadow of that real world." The great scientific revolutionaries of the 1600s went much further—they made the destruction of experience "a basic tenet of philosophical thinking" (ibid.). Beginning with Descartes, Western philosophers have held that the only reliable knowledge is found in the mental states or ideas of our own minds, where we deal with such abstract issues as existence, person, and justice. Everyday experiences such as loving relations and family life, as well as issues of how we should live our day-to-day lives, fell into the realm of disbelief or even disdain. The formative stage of the field of bioethics has evolved within this intellectual heritage, in which both scientific conceptualization and philosophical rationality have functioned at a great distance from the lived experience of ordinary life.

Although a few philosophers after Descartes, notably Thomas Reid, William James, and Stephen Toulmin, have questioned this undermining of our ordinary experiences and practices, over the past twenty years bioethics has been witnessing the rise and convergence of several major schools of thought that seek to retrieve an interpretation of primary moral experience, against the tide of the dominant Western philosophical tradition (Reich 1988, 1990). The linkage between the search for meaning and the study of morality is a major feature of these new developments (Reich 2000). Six of those schools of thought that deserve a new or revised entry in the *EB* are: "pragmatism," "phenomenology," "feminist ethics," and the "ethics of care" (topics that I will discuss in the next two sections), as well as "narrative ethics" and "virtue ethics," especially the virtue ethics that focuses on character and agency.

Other topics, appropriately considered at different levels of bioethical inquiry, deserve mention under the rubric of the turn to experience. A major impetus toward taking experience seriously has been the growing literature that embraces and explains the link between emotions and moral knowledge and judgment while rejecting the traditional view that knowledge arising from experience is unreliable and hence hostile to reason because it is too easily clouded by subjective impulsivity (Nussbaum 1998; Koziak 1999). This philosophical liberation of emotions needs to be linked with a practical articulation of the role of emotions in the practice of medicine (Halpern 2001). The current revival of interest in philosophy as the art of living, which traces back to Socrates and the Stoics (Hadot 1995; Nehamas 1998), also has potential for eventually articulating an experience-based perspective that would be a major component of bioethics theory and practice. The art-of-living sensitivity and philosophy, interwoven with some aspects of virtue, phenomenological, narrative, and care ethics and with social and behavioral aspects of bioethics, are creating a combined intellectual force that is becoming more and more evident in major areas of bioethics like "end-of-life care," "good dying," "care of the aged," "family care," etc., requiring a major recasting of articles in those areas. In addition, attention to experience requires more attention in the *EB* to the use of ethnography and social science analysis of clinical medicine and other areas of bioethics. Finally, it would seem useful if the third edition of *EB* were to discuss the interpretation of primary experience as an organizing theme for bioethics in the articles dealing with the history and methods of ethics and bioethics. When one considers the combined intellectual force of these experience-based approaches and the intellectual and cultural obstacles they all face, one can perhaps see the justification for calling their joint endeavor in bioethics a revolution against millennia of ethical traditions that have been reflected in the dominant approaches to bioethics during its founding period.

A consideration of moral experience as an organizing point for bioethics and the *EB* unavoidably raises the question of postmodernism in bioethics, since experience-based approaches to bioethics accentuate ethical pluralism and generally question the adequacy of a foundational approach that regards principles—and not the interpretation of experience—as the indispensable starting point for ethics. The postmodern critique of ethics holds that foundational approaches to ethics, which claim that universal principles are applicable across cultural and historical differences, are doomed to failure because they are still working with the shards of ethical systems that had intellectual and political power only in the premodern era (Baker 1998a, 1998b; McGrath 1998). Yet not all proponents of experience-based approaches to bioethics share the radical postmodern objections against objectivity, abstraction, universal truth, and universal principles. What is most significant is that the postmodernist critique raises the question of the very possibility of bioethics being pursued effectively in a multicultural world without being submerged in an ineffective relativism or skepticism (Wiesing 1994). The absence of any discussion of postmodern ethics in both the first and second editions of the *EB* must be corrected by inclusion in the third edition of a major entry on "postmodernism" [and bioethics], which would examine not only antifundamentalist theories but the historical, social, and intellectual features of postmodernity itself (Sim 1999); how it has influenced the development of postmodernist theories; how one might critique that worldview; the role of particular moral worldviews; and whether there is the possibility of a new common ethic that can foster moral solidarity while showing regard for primary moral experience in ethics.

Some of the following experientially based approaches to bioethics have never before been discussed separately in *EB*, while others have, but require extensive revisions.

TWO EXPERIENTIAL TOPICS FOR THE *EB*: PHENOMENOLOGY AND PRAGMATISM

One of the greatest obstacles to a consideration of lived moral experience in bioethics, as it is found, for example, in phenomenology, is precisely the dominant agenda of bioethics activity in the United States: public policy making. While some believe that "American bioethics is at its fullest and . . . best" when it helps to produce policy statements by federal and state governments and professional bodies in areas like protection of research subjects and the rights of patients (Jonsen 2001, 44), others may want to claim that other functions of bioethics are more influential and exemplify bioethics at its best, such as bioethics' contribution to the interpretation and understanding of moral meaning—for example, in caregiving, suffering, and professional service—or the enormous impact that bioethics has on education in the sciences, the humanities, and the professions. For the task of creating and maintaining a basic document for the field of bioethics like the *EB*, it really doesn't matter what one thinks is the finest function of bioethicists; what matters most is that all perspectives be given thorough attention. Yet this discussion is important, for at the present time, at least in U.S. culture, it is important to be aware of the seductive nature of policy making and the ways in which it can co-opt intellectual energies in bioethical research, learning, and teaching, with the result that there is little perception of the need for the sort of interpretation offered through phenomenology and related experience-based approaches to bioethics. In carrying out its responsibility to contribute to the integrity of and balance in the field of bioethics, the *EB* should at least create an entry on "phenomenology" and include a discussion of phenomenological method and other comparable approaches to bioethics in the basic articles on ethics and bioethics.

During the first thirty years of the development of bioethics, phenomenology has been largely ignored, in spite of the fact that, more than any other approach to bioethics, it systematically examines the meaning and moral implications of the lived experience of illness, disability, pain and suffering, mental handicap, care, empathy, the therapeutic relationship, and other human experiences related to this discipline. While recent works dealing explicitly with methods in medical bioethics have overlooked the role of phenomenology (Sugarman and Sulmasy 2001), the maturation of methodology in the area of phenomenology in medicine and bioethics is evidenced by the recent appearance of a comprehensive *Handbook of Phenomenology and Medicine* (Toombs 2002). Recent studies in phenomenological approaches to bioethics include Helen Fielding's argument regarding the importance of emotional and noncognitive feedback (including revulsion) when making moral judgments (Fielding 1998) and Michael Daly's analysis of growth in moral wisdom in professional caregivers (Daly 1987). Finally, phenomenologists are confronting radical challenges to their approach, in discussions as to whether phenomenology can function credibly in a postmodernist world that claims the human subject is so decentered that it loses its dignity, or whether, on the contrary, the new particularisms in our society and in moral philosophy in fact are leading us to a new centeredness and a new appreciation of human subjectivity (Visker 1999).

At the end of the nineteenth century, William James and John Dewey spearheaded the efforts of a number of philosophers who were looking for an approach that would reject the dominant disdain for interpreting primary experience of everyday life as a starting point for philosophy (Reed 1996, 18–31). Since the appearance of the second edition of the *EB*, scholars like Glenn McGee (1999), Jonathan Moreno (1999), and Christopher Tollefsen (2000), motivated by a similar philosophical concern, have retrieved the pragmatism of James, Dewey, and others and fashioned the outlines of what they call "pragmatic bioethics." Joseph Fins, Matthew Bacchetta, and Franklin Miller (1997, 1998) have sketched out a method for "clinical pragmatism," and Lynn Jansen (1998) has offered a probing critique of this approach.

Along with phenomenology, feminist ethics, and other approaches that focus on experience, pragmatism distances itself from universal principles, which it regards as theoretical guides or hypotheses regarding desirable outcomes. It also understands moral knowledge as embedded in the world of our experience rather than in a separate realm of abstraction; strives to achieve consensus rather than a final, correct answer; focuses on a process of moral decision making characterized by adaptability and attention to context; and sometimes adopts a Roycean notion of loyalty as a unifying theme. Moreno, who approaches bioethics from the perspective of naturalism, an approach that parallels pragmatism, claims that the dominant American policy-oriented bioethics is and always has been a "Deweyan endeavor": "the naturalistic orientation in bioethics is prevalent but unrecognized . . ." (Moreno 1999, 15). This comment is indicative of the need for a thorough encyclopedia entry that explains and critically evaluates "pragmatism and naturalism" in the entire field of bioethics, not just clinical or policy bioethics.

Discussion of pragmatism leads to a consideration of the thought of German philosopher Jürgen Habermas, who is having a major influence on North American and European ethics. Among the philosophical sources for his "discourse ethics," Habermas employs ideas from pragmatism as well as feminist philosophy, yet he adopts the basic framework of a Kantian theory, endorsing a deontological method pertaining to the presuppositions of discourse. Interestingly, he advocates attention to specific contexts and a balance between cognitive and emotional factors such as empathy and love for neighbor—elements that make his approach useful for both political and bioethical issues. The next edition of the *EB* should discuss Habermas's "discourse ethics" (Habermas 1993), the views of his critics, parallel ideas in "dialogical ethics" (Rehg 1994), and the use of these dialogical methods in bioethics. The influence of Habermas in bioethics raises an interesting organizational question for the *EB*, which has never had entries titled with names of authors; and the question is further accentuated by the rise of interest in grounding an approach to bioethics specifically and directly in the thought of Ludwig Wittgenstein (Elliott 2001).

FEMINIST ETHICS AND THE ETHICS OF CARE: TWO MORE EXPERIENTIAL TOPICS

Over the past twenty years the developing field of feminist ethics has been the most stimulating intellectual component of bioethical discourse, probably because it has been the most powerful instrument for calling moral attention to the morally relevant experiences of individuals and groups that have been passed over in a universalist framework and because it has made the most effective contribution to a critical appraisal of the dominant assumptions of the field while also making substantive contributions to virtually every particular topic within the field. Precisely for these reasons, the task of revising the *EB*'s components of feminist thought is quite complex, because it must take into account an expansive range of methodological and applied topics, must be attentive to an enormous number of significant writers, and must respect the fact that feminist ethics, far from being monolithic, has branched into a variety of schools of thought that are engaged in dialogue with many different types of philosophies and sets of experiences. Consequently, the *EB* must offer a thoroughly re-thought presentation of major entries like "bioethics," "feminist ethics," and "women." In addition, a host of existing topics need to be revised for currency in terms of feminist thought; and new articles need to be created on themes that have emerged recently in feminist ethics.

A good place to start revisiting the entire spectrum of relevant feminist thought is two recently published guides to the field: the first comprehensive reference work dealing with feminist philosophy, edited by Alison Jaggar and Iris Young (1999), and a handbook on feminist bioethics edited by Susan Wolf (1996). It will be important to consider recent developments in some of the main themes that have been pursued in feminist ethics and bioethics from the start: for example, the debate concerning the dominant tradition of moral theory that has made the experience of men the measure of human experience but has claimed universality for the positions it has taken without taking account of women's experience (Benhabib 1995); and the concern that gender blindness conceals the distinct social and political statuses of men and women and hence the very nature of social and political discourse (Fraser 1989). A significant development that should be reflected in the revision of a standard concept like "justice" will show that, whereas a common feminist approach of the 1980s contrasted justice and care quite sharply, one now sees that, largely under feminist influence, some theories of justice include elements, motivations, and justifications in terms of care and compassion, thus replicating to some extent a theme found in the history of ethics from antiquity (Slote 2001). Some of the most important recent work in feminist ethics affecting bioethics has been feminist political philosophy under the leadership of people like Joan C. Tronto (1993). In this tradition, a recent work moves ethics across national borders that have been excessively restrictive for justice-related areas in bioethics, creating the basis for a feminist, multicultural, postcolonial "global bioethics" (Narayan and Harding 2000).

A revised *EB* articulation of feminist bioethics should also take into account recent critiques of feminist ethics and should integrate trends in feminist ethics to which the *EB* and other works in bioethics have paid insufficient attention. Those trends and critiques would urge the following: that more attention be given to religious feminist ethics (Carr and Van Leeuwen 1996), the work of black feminists (Collins 2000), the insights of Hispanic American women (Isasi-Díaz 1996), and European scholars' work on gendered meanings in philosophy (Nagl-Docekal and Klinger 2000). Among the critiques that have been published recently regarding feminist philosophy, the revision of a central document in bioethics should take into account arguments for historical correctives regarding basic ideas in feminism (Jouve 1998) and the critiques of the relationship of U.S. feminist theory to the Western liberal tradition (Jamieson 2001). Finally, the *EB* should introduce entries and/or articles within entries on topics suggested by feminist discussions, for example: "moral agency," "gender," and "mothering and fathering," to mention but a few.

The ethics of care has taken a major turn, in the sense that its intellectual boundaries are no longer so strongly defined by its feminist origins. The ethics of care has stimulated nonfeminists to embrace feminist care-ideas as a corrective to the faults in their own ethical theories; and it increasingly grounds itself in all sorts of contemporary and historical frames of reference. The *EB* must show how feminist thought on care continues to grow and to have an enormous influence in many areas affecting bioethics; but it must also demonstrate how care is now standing on its own as a distinctive idea in the larger history of ideas—a historical accomplishment that would not have taken place had it not been for twentieth-century feminist thought.

The new era of the ethics of care that the *EB* has the task of defining is characterized, first of all, by the careful work of scholars who are offering a strong intellectual grounding for care in the moral life, in moral philosophy, and in professional settings, thus belying earlier criticism that care theory was in a state of chaos. For example, Patricia Benner attempts to establish a moral-philosophical grounding for care ethics by placing it in careful dialogue with both Greek and Judeo-Christian virtue ethics; and she spells out the implications in her dialogue between nursing and medicine, thus building substantial bridges between the ethics of the two professions (Benner 1997). Relying on ideas drawn from eighteenth-century moral sentimentalism and the motive of "caring" derived from a recent "feminine" morality of caring to which he assigns an expanded role, Michael Slote develops a virtue ethics from which he argues for a general account of right and wrong action as well as social justice (Slote 2001). Stan van Hooft draws on Heidegger and Lévinas for an understanding of care as an ontological structure of human existence, arguing that ethics has more to do with the social forms of caring for ourselves and others than with obligations (van Hooft 1995)—an approach that he has also applied to bioethics (van Hooft 1996). On the other hand, Peta Bowden takes issue with accounts of the ethics of care that focus on alleged basic principles, arguing instead for an interpretation of caring practices, which she organizes around four models: mothering, friendship, nursing, and citizenship (Bowden 1997).

The ethics of care continues to be used extensively in applied areas, for example, in "medical ethics" (Rhodes 1995), "environmental ethics" (King 1996), "animal ethics" (Donovan 1996), and the ethics of "pharmacy," which has been radically reoriented by ideas of care and covenant (Haddad and Buerki 1996). As care of the sick, especially the chronically ill, shifts from hospital to home, "family care" becomes an important new topic for the field of bioethics (Nelson and Nelson 1995).

The *EB* will have to pay particular attention to the growing literature on political aspects of care: for example, whether the idea of care creates gender inequality (Harrington 1999), and how justice and care are interrelated (Clement 1996). It would also be interesting to present in one place the historical antecedents to which the care ethics literature appeals, for example, Heidegger's ethic of care. Since the idea of care challenges the primacy if not exclusivity accorded to the idea of "beneficence/benevolence" in bioethics, the *EB* should discuss other care-ideas—virtues, principles, motivations, and themes of social ethos that have served approximately the same purposes as care and beneficence in previous historical eras. This should be done not only for historical reasons, but also because most of the following are reappearing in literature dealing with medical theory, nursing theory, medical bioethics, and environmental bioethics: "sympathy," a very important topic with a longer and stronger moral lineage than either compassion or empathy (Donovan 1996), "hospitality," "stewardship," "friendship," "charity," "covenant," and "altruism."

Vulnerability: A Thematic Topic That Could Change the Shape of Bioethics

I believe there are three thematic topics that could substantially alter the shape of bioethics over the next decade. At the very least, if taken seriously, they could prompt a thoroughgoing reevaluation of the field. Interestingly, none of the three have appeared in previous editions of the *EB*. They are "vulnerability," "religion," and "globalization."

Although vulnerability has rarely been the object of bioethical inquiry and certainly has never been discussed in the *EB*, it may well turn out to be the most significant bioethical idea of the next era. The issuance of the 1998 Barcelona Declaration, which culminated a three-year study for the European Commission, has given a "principle of vulnerability" international recognition in the field of bioethics by recommending that it be one of four major principles for bioethics discourse (Barcelona Declaration 2000). The two volumes of papers on the European principles of bioethics show that a new attentiveness to primary human experience is currently highlighting the salience for bioethics of the idea that humans are vulnerable—literally meaning susceptible to being wounded or, figuratively, to being harmed—and, consequently, are dependent and live in a situation of interdependence (Rendtorff and Kemp 2000; Kemp, Rendtorff, and Johansen 2000). A great variety of characteristics shape the condition called vulnerability: dependency, fragility, and relative defenselessness in those conditions; susceptibility to harm and actually being harmed; susceptibility to suffering and actual suffering; etc. Vulnerabilities may be biological (corporeal), psychological and spiritual, social, environmental, or cultural, all of which have significance for contemporary bioethics.

Contemporary philosophy is increasingly regarding vulnerability as part of the basic identity of all humans who, because of their own vulnerability and dependency as well as that of others, have the constant characteristic of needing care (by self, others, and society) and the moral responsibility to respond to the vulnerability of others. For example, Emmanuel Lévinas defines vulnerability as intrinsic to human subjectivity, constituting the self as ethical subject and motivating the moral imperative to take responsibility for the other (Lévinas 1969). For Jürgen Habermas, vulnerability is the foundation of the notions of care, responsibility, and empathy; and profound vulnerability is the basis of ethics (Rendtorff and Kemp 2000, 48–49). In Paul Ricoeur's philosophy, vulnerability means that we must live with mortality and take care of the other as a fragile subject (Rendtorff and Kemp 2000, 49–50). Alasdair MacIntyre, correcting a fundamental error in his earlier work on virtue, argues for the fundamental role played by virtues needed to respond to vulnerability and disability in ourselves and in others (MacIntyre 1999, 5). Feminist philosophy has been instrumental in bringing the notion of vulnerability to bear on moral philosophy; for example, Okin argues that the disproportionate vulnerabilities of women and children in the gendered models of family and society that are used by John Rawls create flaws in his theory of justice (Okin 1989). Rejecting the adequacy of the liberal contractualist ethic between autonomous strangers, care theorist Virginia Held holds that the starting point for public ethics should be mutual dependency in the context of an interconnected social reality that one sees, for example, in the care of infants and of those who care for infants (Held 1999). In addition, two issues of *Hypatia* (vol. 16, no. 4; vol. 17, no. 3) are devoted to the experience of and moral issues related to disability.

Vulnerability has been a significant theme in political philosophy for some time. For example, Robert Goodin offers a consequentialist argument regarding special and general welfare responsibilities to protect the vulnerable (Goodin 1985); and for Judith Shklar, rights are tools for protecting all vulnerable persons in a community, specifically by limiting cruelty and the fear of cruelty (Shklar 1986). Shklar's insistence that rights are for the sake of the weakest and feeblest among us is reminiscent of the Jewish moral law that requires care for the most vulnerable, beginning with widows and orphans and including the poor and strangers—a moral mandate that is also characteristic of Christian and Muslim ethics (Avery-Peck 2000). Thus, properly conceived, the notion of vulnerability could be applied to bioethics from perspectives as varied as phenomenology,

Aristotelian moral philosophy, feminist philosophy, American political philosophy, and the ethics of the principal religious traditions.

Occasional earlier works on the idea/principle of vulnerability in bio-ethics—by Potter (1971), Reich (1993), Campbell (1994), and Pellegrino and Thomasma (1997, 54–66)—contain the seeds for further development, but did not, of themselves, result in a wide recognition of the principle and moral idea of vulnerability in bioethics. Yet it is now being proposed that the principle of vulnerability belongs to the most essential principles in bioethics and biolaw (Rendtorff and Kemp 2000). The implications of an ethic of vulnerability for bioethics are far-reaching: they suggest that the value of autonomy should be placed in the context of care for others instead of vice versa (Rendtorff and Kemp 2000); that the notion of equality in theories of justice must be rethought because of the centrality of our experience of dependency (Kittay 1999); that due to the thinness of the abstract principles of nonmaleficence and beneficence in contemporary analytic bioethics, these principles should be replaced with a more richly responsive virtue of concerned care (MacIntyre 1999); and that all approaches to environmental, social, research, nursing, and medical bioethics should be rethought in light of the ideas of vulnerability and dependency. The next edition of the *EB* should certainly include a major article on vulnerability (linked with the idea of "dependency") and should include a discussion of it in entries on many other topics.

RELIGION: A SECOND THEMATIC TOPIC THAT COULD CHANGE THE SHAPE OF BIOETHICS

One of the most important topics for the next era of bioethics will be the role of religion and religious ideas in bioethics discourse. This claim will not easily be accepted, for several reasons. Although it is commonly acknowledged that ethics rests on two legs of the humanities—philosophical and religious sources—less attention has been paid to theological and religious ethics in the past decade of bioethics perhaps than ever before. Panels are convened in the U.S. to hear "religious views" on issues like stem cell research and cloning; but the intention seems formally representative and the interest largely restricted to the level of achieving a consensus in a pluralistic culture on one or two policy-related options. Furthermore, several generations of bioethicists lack a robust familiarity with the religious meanings and arguments with which they are dealing. This is not surprising: Since the Enlightenment the goal has been to remove all religious "myths" so that a myth-free science could rule human rational life; and as societies evolve, it was assumed that science would remain in the ascendancy and religion would simply fall away. However, as Jean Bethke Elshtain has pointed out (Religion and . . . 2001), it has not worked out that way. Religions are having an enormous impact on political events and the search for social justice; and people are turning more and more to religious and spiritual sources for a sense of meaning in areas of life pertaining to bioethics. I suspect that changes in religious ideas will have far more impact on the bioethics of the next period than changes in science.

My own view is that if the *EB* is to serve the field of bioethics well, it must make major adjustments in how it approaches topics related to religion, religious ethics, religious influence in bioethics, and the many contemporary spiritualities that are not formally linked with the teachings of religious bodies. While building on the considerable strengths of past editions, the next edition should (1) acknowledge the growing relevance of the distinction between religious orthodoxy and religious orthopraxis— i.e., that practices and their interpretation, and not just formally correct religious teachings, manifest the ethics of religious moral traditions. It should also (2) expand its coverage beyond the religious ethics that aligns itself closely with (or critiques) formal teachings of religions to include the constructive work of rational theological inquiry in bioethics; and (3) offer a sociological analysis of the power of religious authority in bioethics, for example, the historically conditioned political power of institutional Islamic and Roman Catholic influence in bioethics policies in various parts of the world. It should (4) provide explanations of how religions, in their scriptures and formal teachings as well as in the belief systems of their adherents, have supported the violence that wounds as well as the care that heals, especially in the fundamentalist context of the past century and a half—and the implications of this dark side of religion. It should (5) review the ideas currently being offered on whether and how secular ethics differs from religious ethics and the significance of the reliance of leading moral philosophers like Rawls on intuitions based in religious moral traditions; (6) examine whether and to what extent the recent literature on "science and religion" has a bearing on bioethics; and (7) provide a careful analysis of the postmodernist elements of and critiques of religious bioethics, as well as attitudes toward postmodernism in religious bioethics. It will be especially important to discuss the contrast between bioethical writings that utilize a negative, skeptical view of postmodernism to portray religious and theological bioethics in a "nonecumenical" way that restricts their significance to a fundamentalist stance, while many theological ethicists and even entire religious groups acknowledge that they function in a pluralistic world and accept major aspects of a second, more positive postmodernism (Westphal 2001). Bioethics needs to catch up with the current, vital resurgence of religious studies; and the *EB* needs to acknowledge more clearly the strong contributions currently being made by religious bioethicists (Davis and Zoloth 1999).

GLOBALIZATION: A THIRD THEMATIC TOPIC THAT COULD CHANGE THE SHAPE OF BIOETHICS

The phenomena of economic, financial, social, political, and moral globalization and the issues it raises are profoundly altering bioethics. Two of the principal reasons why globalization can be expected to change the shape of bioethics are (1) because globalization in a post-sovereign world shifts a significant weight of the agency of responsible health care from individuals who care for health (professionals, family members, self), other contractual agents, and public agencies to entire nations, international governments, nongovernmental organizations, industries, and churches; and (2) because globalization alters our assumptions about the object of care, extending it to all humans including the world's neediest.

Ethical issues regarding disease, famine, and poverty raised by contemporary globalization and transnationalism include the basic question whether there is a moral responsibility on the part of states or other international actors such as multinational pharmaceutical firms toward members of political communities beyond the frontiers of their own sovereign territories or independent organizations. Kantians, communitarians, and other theorists that debate the nature and location of the moral conduct of states tend to work within boundaries of a justice defined in terms of territorial sovereignty (Beitz 1979). On the other hand, in the past decade there has been a growing interest among "anti-foundationalist" scholars who draw on continental philosophers to argue for a "de-territorialized" responsibility for the marginal, the dispossessed, and the vulnerable who are silenced by or do not fit into the moral logic of the territorial state (Campbell and Shapiro 1999). Similarly, feminist scholars working in international relations speak of "empathetic cooperation" as a mode of transnational care for the Other (Sylvester 1994), while other scholars seek social justice through globalization even at the expense of restraining nationalism (Kitching 2001). The *EB* needs to capture this new ethical vision.

Other issues raised by globalization for bioethics include these important questions: how globalization, with its short-term, sometimes exploitative actions, adversely affects the health of humans and nonhuman living things; how globalization might be used to improve the health of humans and nonhumans through long-term, health-sustaining programs; and how to formulate these questions and appropriate responses to them. To do this properly requires taking into account all the disciplines and organizations that pertain to bioethics in the global setting. A major example is found in controversies regarding relief of the AIDS crisis in Africa on the part of the pharmaceutical industry, nations, NGOs, and churches. There appears to be a need to take a critical look at the ways in which these debates are shaped by first-world economic principles, state interests, and ethical assumptions about distribution of goods, moneys, and products. For example, the first-world assumptions that shape the currently dominant ethical agenda in this area—that poverty causes AIDS, that condoms and not changes in primary sexual behavior are the only behavioral solution for Africans, that antiretroviral drugs should be supplied without massive prior attention to infrastructural distributional needs, and that disproportional health spending on AIDS is justified— are all currently being called into question on the basis of sociological and anthropological studies.[5] The *EB* needs to provide a careful and thorough examination of globalization and global health problems from an interdisciplinary perspective.

In addition to addressing the issues of globalization, the *EB* should turn its attention to special issues touching on what is now called "global bioethics," which has two distinct meanings. The first, more mainstream, use of the term focuses on concerns with the application of universal, concrete bioethical standards and/or principles worldwide. Thus, while Ruth Macklin defends the global use of fundamental principles (Macklin 1998), opponents argue that universal principles cannot be used to form a useful foundation for a global ethics (Takala 2001; Engelhardt 1998). The second definition of "global bioethics," which is particular to the late Van Rensselaer Potter, has humanity's survival as its goal and requires decisions regarding environmental care and health care (Jameton 1994).

Finally, there is the issue of "globalism in the exchange of bioethical ideas," which should be discussed and even implemented in the *EB*. Among the current critiques of U.S. bioethics one finds a criticism of U.S. hegemony in international bioethics (Garrafa 2001). I believe the *EB* can do at least two things to help establish some of the conditions for a more globalist exchange of bioethical ideas. First, it should include articles on "indigenous" bioethical approaches that have been developed in all parts of the world, organized conceptually (not just geographically) and *placed side by side* with U.S. and other first-world bioethical frameworks. Second, it would seem advisable to invite European or Latin American scholars, including women, to prepare the major articles on the traditional principles of bioethics that have been developed within the United States, as a way of strengthening these "standard" articles with contributions of ideas from foreign-language sources as well as a critique from other cultures—contributions that U.S. scholars are generally not capable of making. An action of this sort could also have the effect of widening the boundaries of what is regarded as the intellectual "center" of bioethics and in this way expanding global bioethical dialogue.

CONCLUSION

My thirty-two-year engagement with the *EB* prompts a few general comments regarding passions and sentiments that mobilize work in bioethics and become ingredient in it. I would suggest that an intellectual passion (in my case, a passion for the intellectual implications of moral experience and interpretation) is not only allowable but quite possibly indispensable for pursuing a work such as I have described, especially in the interests of perceiving issues that might otherwise escape one's attention. Of course, in the end, a passion of this sort must be tempered by a strong sense of "objectivity" and fairness in actually structuring a reference work like the *EB*. An overarching sentiment that has dominated my work of shepherding the *EB* has been the constant feeling of responsibility for building and maintaining in good quality the central document of the field by gathering together and developing a close collaborative relationship with a host of people smarter than I. Finally, there has been the gradually emerging sentiment that it has all been an experience of care—caring about the whole field of bioethics and taking care of this one hopefully reliable articulation of that field.

ACKNOWLEDGMENTS

I would like to acknowledge, with gratitude, the support of the Lilly Endowment, Inc., for the Project on the History of Care, which enabled me to prepare the portions of this chapter dealing with the principle of vulnerability and the ethics of care. I am also grateful to the Plunkett Centre for Ethics in Health Care at St. Vincent's Hospital in Sydney, Australia, and to the Australian Catholic University, whose generous offer of a visiting professorship made it possible for me to finalize the drafting of this essay. In addition, I want to express my appreciation for the assistance of Peter Mandaville, Jeremy Snyder, and Randy Wheeler in gathering information used in this essay.

Notes

1. Evaluation of the role and function of the *Encyclopedia of Bioethics*, Daniel Callahan, 1989.

2. The editors' areas of responsibility were as follows: Dan Beauchamp (Public Health Bioethics); Arthur Caplan (Organ Transplantation and Biomedical Technology); Christine Cassell (Health Care and Health Care Systems); James F. Childress and Stanley Hauerwas (Fundamental Concepts and Principles); Allen R. Dyer (Mental Health, Behavioral Issues, and Sexuality); John C. Fletcher (Genetics); Albert R. Jonsen (History of Medical Ethics; World Religions); Patricia King (Reproductive Technologies); Loretta Kopelman (Research Ethics); Ruth Purtilo (Professional Ethics and the Professional-Patient Relationship); Holmes Rolston III (Environmental Bioethics and Animal Bioethics); Robert M. Veatch (Death and Dying); and Donald P. Warwick (Population Bioethics).

3. Stephen Post, who served as the second edition's associate editor, working directly with the editor-in-chief, is editor-in-chief of the third edition. I have deliberately not consulted with him or his editorial colleagues in the preparation of this essay, lest there be a reciprocal influence that might prejudice the results of the findings that I offer here.

4. I am grateful to the staff of the National Reference Center for Bioethics Literature at the Kennedy Institute of Ethics at Georgetown University for their consultation and advice in the preparation of this essay, particularly in reference to topics that are currently emerging in bioethics literature. I am especially indebted to Doris Goldstein (Director), Joy Kahn, Pat McCarrick, Martina Darragh, and Laura Bishop. For over thirty years the *EB* project and I have always been able to count on the exceptional range of knowledge and exemplary devotion to the communication of information of the staff of the Bioethics Information Retrieval Project, under the founding leadership of LeRoy Walters.

5. Personal communication from Edward C. Green, Ph.D., Harvard School of Public Health.

References

Avery-Peck, Alan J. 2000. Charity in Judaism. *The Encyclopaedia of Judaism*. Vol. I. Leiden/Boston/Köln: Brill.

Baker, Robert. 1998a. A Theory of International Bioethics: Multiculturalism, Postmodernism, and the Bankruptcy of Fundamentalism. *Kennedy Institute of Ethics Journal* 8(3): 201–31.

———. 1998b. A Theory of International Bioethics: The Negotiable and the Non-Negotiable. *Kennedy Institute of Ethics Journal,* 8(3): 233–73.

Barcelona Declaration. 2000. In *Basic Ethical Principles in European Bioethics and Biolaw*. Vol. I: *Autonomy, Dignity, Integrity, and Vulnerability* by Jacob Dahl

Rendtorff and Peter Kemp. Report to the European Commission of the BIOMED-II Project, "Basic Ethical Principles in Bioethics and Biolaw 1995–1998." Copenhagen: Centre for Ethics and Law; Barcelona: Institut Borja de Bioètica.

Beauchamp, Dan E., and Bonnie Steinbock, eds. 1999. *New Ethics for the Public's Health*. New York: Oxford University Press.

Beitz, Charles. 1979. *Political Theory and International Relations*. Princeton, N.J.: Princeton University Press.

Benhabib, Seyla. 1995. The Debate over Women and Moral Theory Revisited. In *Feminists Read Habermas: Gendering the Subject of Discourse*, edited by Johanna Meehan. New York: Routledge.

Benner, Patricia. 1984. *From Novice to Expert: Excellence and Power in Clinical Nursing Practice*. Menlo Park, Calif.: Addison-Wesley.

———. 1997. A Dialogue between Virtue Ethics and Care Ethics. *Theoretical Medicine* 18(1–2): 47–61.

Bowden, Peta. 1997. *Caring: Gender-Sensitive Ethics*. New York: Routledge.

Campbell, Alastair V. 1994. Dependency: The Foundational Value in Medical Ethics. In *Medicine and Moral Reasoning*, edited by K. W. M. Fulford. New York: Cambridge University Press.

Campbell, David, and Michael J. Shapiro, eds. 1999. *Moral Spaces: Rethinking Ethics and World Politics*. Minneapolis: University of Minnesota Press.

Carr, Anne, and Mary Stewart Van Leeuwen, eds. 1996. *Religion, Feminism, and the Family*. Louisville, Ky.: Westminster John Knox.

Christie, Dolores L., Dena S. Davis, and Sumner B. Twiss. 1996. Review of *Encyclopedia of Bioethics*, Rev. ed. *Religious Studies Review* 22(4): 279–92.

Clement, Grace. 1996. *Care, Autonomy, and Justice: Feminism and the Ethic of Care*. Boulder, Colo.: Westview Press.

Collins, Patricia Hill. 2000. *Black Feminist Thought: Knowledge, Consciousness, and the Politics of Empowerment*. Rev. ed. New York: Routledge.

Daly, Michael E. 1987. Towards a Phenomenology of Caregiving: Growth in the Caregiver Is a Vital Component. *Journal of Medical Ethics* 13: 34–39.

Davis, Dena S., and Laurie Zoloth, eds., 1999. *Notes from a Narrow Ridge: Religion and Bioethics*. Hagerstown, Md.: University Publishing Group.

Donovan, Josephine. 1996. Attention to Suffering: A Feminist Caring Ethic for the Treatment of Animals. *Journal of Social Philosophy* 27(1): 81–102.

Elliott, Carl, ed. 2001. *Slow Cures and Bad Philosophers: Essays on Wittgenstein, Medicine, and Bioethics*. Durham, N.C.: Duke University Press.

Engelhardt, H. Tristram, Jr. 1998. Critical Care: Why There Is No Global Bioethics. *Journal of Medicine and Philosophy* 23(6): 643–51.

Fielding, Helen A. 1998. Body Measures: Phenomenological Considerations of Corporeal Ethics. *Journal of Medicine and Philosophy* 23(5): 533–45.

Fins, Joseph J., Matthew D. Bacchetta, and Franklin G. Miller. 1997. Clinical Pragmatism: A Method of Moral Problem Solving. *Kennedy Institute of Ethics Journal* 7(2): 129–45.

Fins, Joseph J., Franklin G. Miller, and Matthew D. Bacchetta. 1998. Clinical Pragmatism: Bridging Theory and Practice. *Kennedy Institute of Ethics Journal* 8(1): 37–42.

Fraser, Nancy. 1989. *Unruly Practices: Power, Discourse, and Gender in Contemporary Social Theory.* Minneapolis: University of Minnesota Press.

Garrafa, Volnei. 2001. Current Panorama of Bioethics in Brazil. *IAB News: The Newsletter of the International Association of Bioethics* 12: 5–9.

Goodin, Robert. 1985. *Protecting the Vulnerable: A Reanalysis of Our Social Responsibilities.* Chicago: University of Chicago Press.

Gostin, Lawrence O. 2000. *Public Health Law: Power, Duty, Restraint.* Berkeley: University of California Press; New York: Milbank Memorial Fund.

Habermas, Jürgen. 1993. *Justification and Application: Remarks on Discourse Ethics.* Translated by Claran Cronin. Cambridge, Mass.: MIT Press.

Haddad, Amy Marie, and Robert A. Buerki, eds. 1996. *Ethical Dimensions of Pharmaceutical Care.* Binghamton, N.Y.: Pharmaceutical Products Press.

Hadot, Pierre. 1995. *Philosophy as a Way of Life: Spiritual Exercises from Socrates to Foucault.* Edited with an introduction by Arnold I. Davidson. Translated by Michael Chase. Oxford, U.K., and Cambridge, Mass.: Blackwell.

Halpern, Jodi. 2001. *From Detached Concern to Empathy: Humanizing Medical Practice.* Oxford and New York: Oxford University Press.

Harrington, Mona. 1999. *Care and Equality.* New York: Knopf.

Held, Virginia. 1999. Liberalism and the Ethics of Care. In *On Feminist Ethics and Politics*, edited by Claudia Card. Lawrence: University Press of Kansas.

Hottois, Gilbert, ed. 2001. *Nouvelle encyclopedie de bioethique.* Bruxelles: De Boeck.

Isasi-Díaz, Ada Maria. 1996. *Mujerista Theology: A Theology for the Twenty-first Century.* Maryknoll, N.Y.: Orbis.

Jaggar, Alison, and Iris Young, eds. 1999. *Companion to Feminist Philosophy.* Walden, Mass.: Blackwell.

Jameton, Andrew. 1994. Global Bioethics. *Cambridge Quarterly of Healthcare Ethics* 3(3): 449–51.

Jamieson, Beth Kiyoko. 2001. *Real Choice: Feminism, Freedom, and the Limits of Law.* University Park: Penn State University Press.

Jansen, Lynn A. 1998. Assessing Clinical Pragmatism. *Kennedy Institute of Ethics Journal* 8(1): 23–36.

Jonsen, Albert R. 2001. Beating Up Bioethics. *Hastings Center Report* 31(5): 40–45.

Jouve, Nicole Ward. 1998. *Female Genesis: Creativity, Self, and Gender.* New York: St. Martin's Press.

Kemp, Peter, Jacob Rendtorff, and Niels Mattsson Johansen, eds. 2000. *Bioethics and Biolaw, Volume 2: Four Ethical Principles.* Copenhagen: Rhodos International Science and Art Publishers and Centre for Ethics and Law.

King, Robert J. H. 1996. Caring about Nature: Feminist Ethics and the Environment. In *Ecological Feminist Philosophies,* edited by Karen J. Warren. Bloomington: Indiana University Press.

Kirkengen, Anna Luise. 2001. *Inscribed Bodies: Health Impact of Childhood Sexual Abuse.* Dordrecht and Boston: Kluwer Academic.

Kitching, Gavin. 2001. *Seeking Social Justice through Globalization: Escaping a Nationalist Perspective.* University Park: Penn State University Press.

Kittay, Eva. 1999. *Love's Labor: Essays on Women, Equality, and Dependence.* New York: Routledge.

Koczwara, Bogda M., and Timothy J. Madigan. 1997. The Heterogeneity of Clinical Ethics: The State of the Field as Reflected in the *Encyclopedia of Bioethics. The Journal of Medicine and Philosophy* 22: 75–88.

Korff, Wilhelm, ed. 1998. *Lexikon der Bioethik.* Gütersloh: Gütersloher Verlagshaus.

Koziak, Barbara. 1999. *Retrieving Political Emotion: Thumos, Aristotle, and Gender.* University Park: Penn State University Press.

Lévinas, Emmanuel. 1969 (1961). *Totality and Infinity.* Translated by Alphonso Lingis. The Hague: Nijhoff; Pittsburgh: Duquesne.

MacIntyre, Alasdair. 1999. *Dependent Rational Animals: Why Human Beings Need the Virtues.* Chicago: Open Court.

Macklin, Ruth. 1998. A Defense of Fundamental Principles and Human Rights: A Reply to Robert Baker. *Kennedy Institute of Ethics Journal* 8(4): 403–22.

Mahowald, Mary Briody. 1993. *Women and Children in Health Care: An Unequal Majority.* New York: Oxford University Press.

Mayeroff, Milton. 1971. *On Caring.* New York: HarperCollins.

McGee, Glenn. 1999. Pragmatic Method and Bioethics. *Pragmatic Bioethics,* edited by Glenn McGee. Nashville: Vanderbilt University Press.

McGrath, Pam. 1998. Autonomy, Discourse, and Power: A Postmodern Reflection on Principlism and Bioethics. *Journal of Medicine and Philosophy* 23(5): 516–32.

Michel, Sonya. 1999. *Children's Interests/Mother's Rights: The Shaping of America's Child Policy.* New Haven, Conn.: Yale University Press.

Moreno, Jonathan. 1999. Bioethics Is a Naturalism. In *Pragmatic Bioethics,* edited by Glenn McGee. Nashville: Vanderbilt University Press.

Murray, Thomas H. 1996. *The Worth of a Child.* Berkeley: University of California Press.

Nagl-Docekal, Herda, and Cornelia Klinger, eds. 2000. *Continental Philosophy in Feminist Perspective: Re-Reading the Canon in German.* University Park: Penn State University Press.

Narayan, Uma, and Sandra Harding, eds. 2000. *Decentering the Center: Philosophy for a Multicultural, Postcolonial, and Feminist World*. Bloomington: Indiana University Press.

Nehamas, Alexander. 1998. *The Art of Living: Socratic Reflections from Plato to Foucault*. Berkeley: University of California Press.

Nelson, Hilde Lindemann, and James Lindemann Nelson. 1995. *The Patient in the Family: An Ethics of Medicine and Families*. New York: Routledge.

Nussbaum, Martha C. 1998. Morality and Emotions. In *Routledge Encyclopedia of Philosophy*, edited by Edward Craig. Vol. VI. London: Routledge.

Okin, Susan Moller. 1989. *Justice, Gender, and the Family*. New York: Basic Books.

Pellegrino, Edmund D., and David C. Thomasma. 1997. *Helping and Healing: Religious Commitment in Health Care*. Washington, D.C.: Georgetown University Press.

Potter, Van Rensselaer. 1971. *Bioethics: Bridge to the Future*. Englewood Cliffs, N.J.: Prentice Hall.

Reed, Edward S. 1996. *The Necessity of Experience*. New Haven, Conn., and London: Yale University Press.

Rehg, William. 1994. *Insight and Solidarity: A Study in the Discourse Ethics of Jürgen Habermas*. Berkeley: University of California Press.

Reich, Warren T., ed. 1978. *Encyclopedia of Bioethics*. 4 volumes. New York: Macmillan, Free Press.

———. 1988. Experiential Ethics as a Foundation for Dialogue between Health Communication and Health-Care Ethics. *Journal of Applied Communication Research* 16(1): 16–28.

———. 1990. Ein neues Paradigma: Erfahrung als Quelle der Bioethik. In *Ethik in den Wissenschaften: Ariadnefaden im technischen Labyrinth?* edited by Klaus Steigleder and Dietmar Mieth. Tübingen: Attempto.

———. 1993. Alle origini dell'etica medica: Mito del contratto o mito di Cura? In *Modelli di Medicina: Crisi e Attualità dell'Idea di Professione*, edited by P. Cattorini and R. Mordacci. Milan: Europa Scienze Umane Editrice.

———, ed. 1995. *Encyclopedia of Bioethics*. Revised edition. 5 volumes. New York: Simon & Schuster Macmillan.

———. 2000. The Search for Moral Meaning: A New Era for Bioethics. In *Bioethics and Biolaw*, Vol. I: *Judgement of Life*, edited by Peter Kemp, Jacob Rendtorff, and Niels Matsson Johansen. Copenhagen: Rhodos International Science and Art Publishers & Centre for Ethics and Law.

Religion and . . . : A Public Intellectual and Her Many Projects. 2001. *News of the National Humanities Center* (winter): 1–3.

Rendtorff, Jacob Dahl, and Peter Kemp, 2000. *Basic Ethical Principles in European Bioethics and Biolaw*. Vol. I: *Autonomy, Dignity, Integrity, and Vulnerability*. Report to the European Commission of the BIOMED-II Project, "Basic Ethical

Principles in Bioethics and Biolaw 1995–1998." Copenhagen: Centre for Ethics and Law; Barcelona: Institut Borja de Bioètica.

Rhodes, Rosamond. 1995. Love Thy Patient: Justice, Caring, and the Doctor-Patient Relationship. *Cambridge Quarterly for Healthcare Ethics* 4(4): 434–47.

Schenck, David, Glenn C. Graber, and Charles H. Reynolds. 1981. Review of *Encyclopedia of Bioethics*. *Religious Studies Review* 7(1): 5–14.

Shklar, Judith. 1986. Injustice, Injury, and Inequality: An Introduction. In *Justice and Equality Here and Now*, edited by Frank Lucash. Ithaca, N.Y.: Cornell University Press.

Sim, Stuart, ed. 1999. *The Routledge Critical Dictionary of Postmodern Thought*. New York: Routledge.

Slote, Michael. 2001. *Morals from Motives*. New York: Oxford University Press.

Steinfels, Peter. 1979. From Abortion to Zygote Banking (Review of *Encyclopedia of Bioethics*). *Hastings Center Report* 9(3): 40–41.

Stolk, Joop, Theo A. Boer, and Ruth Seldenrijk, eds. 2000. *Meaningful Care: A Multidisciplinary Approach to the Meaning of Care for People with Mental Retardation*. Dordrecht and Boston: Kluwer.

Sugarman, Jeremy, and Daniel P. Sulmasy, eds. 2001. *Methods in Medical Ethics*. Washington, D.C.: Georgetown University Press.

Sylvester, Christine. 1994. *Feminist Theory and International Relations in a Postmodern Era*. Cambridge, U.K.: Cambridge University Press.

Takala, Tuija. 2001. What Is Wrong with Global Bioethics? On the Limitations of the Four Principles Approach. *Cambridge Quarterly of Healthcare Ethics* 10(1): 72–77.

ten Have, Henk, ed. 1992. *Ethiek & Recht in de Gezondheidszorg*. Supplements: 1995, 1998, 2000. Deventer: Kluwer.

Tollefsen, Christopher. 2000. What Would John Dewey Do? The Promises and Perils of Pragmatic Bioethics. *Journal of Medicine and Philosophy* 25(1): 77–106.

Toombs, Kay, ed. 2002. *Handbook of Phenomenology and Medicine*. Dordrecht, Holland, and Boston, Mass.: Kluwer Academic.

Tronto, Joan C. 1993. *Moral Boundaries: A Political Argument for an Ethic of Care*. New York: Routledge.

van Hooft, Stan. 1995. *Caring: An Essay in the Philosophy of Ethics*. Foreword by Jean Watson. Niwot: University Press of Colorado.

———. 1996. Bioethics and Caring. *Journal of Medical Ethics* 22(2): 83–89.

Visker, Rudi. 1999. *Truth and Singularity: Taking Foucault into Phenomenology*. Dordrecht, Holland, and Boston, Mass.: Kluwer Academic.

Warren, Karen J., ed. 1996. *Feminist Philosophies*. Bloomington: Indiana University Press.

Westphal, Merold. 2001. *Overcoming Onto-Theology: Toward a Postmodern Christian Faith*. New York: Fordham University Press.

Wiesing, Urban. 1994. Style and Responsibility: Medicine in Postmodernity. *Theoretical Medicine* 15(3): 277–90.

Wolf, Susan M., ed. 1996. *Feminism and Bioethics: Beyond Reproduction*. New York: Oxford University Press.

10

The Dangers of Difference, Revisited

PATRICIA A. KING

Thirty years ago, in late July 1972, Associated Press reporter Jean Heller broke the story of the longest and most scandalous "non-therapeutic" experiment on human beings in U.S. history. Beginning in Macon County, Alabama, in 1932, the United States Public Health Service (USPHS) had been conducting the "Tuskegee Study of Untreated Syphilis in the Negro Male"—a forty-year study of untreated syphilis involving 399 poor black men suffering from the disease and 201 control subjects.

The seminal account of the USPHS-sponsored study is given by James Jones in his book *Bad Blood* (Jones 1993). As Jones describes, this was a "study in nature" intended to track the effects of untreated syphilis on black humans over time. The research subjects[1] were misled about the nature and intent of the study, and therefore informed consent was impossible. When, in the 1940s, penicillin was discovered to be a cure for syphilis, the monitoring physicians of the Tuskegee Syphilis Study did not give their subjects the treatment—indeed, the researchers took measures to prevent other physicians from giving the needed drug.

The Tuskegee Syphilis Study was not an aberration, as African Americans were extensively used as the subjects of medical experimentation during the nineteenth century (Byrd and Clayton 2000). Rather, the study can be seen as one chapter in the long history of still-extant racial ideologies and practices in U.S. science and medicine. The Tuskegee Syphilis Study has, however, attained a special status. As Susan Reverby points out in the introduction to her influential book *Tuskegee's Truths*, "[t]he Tuskegee Study is America's metaphor for racism in medical research" (Reverby 2000, 3). As Reverby makes clear, there are many dimensions to the study, each emphasizing different aspects of the multifaceted interactions between researchers and their subjects and even between science itself and the culture in which it flourishes. Interestingly, even though much has been written about the Tuskegee Syphilis Study, bioethicists have largely failed to explore the impact of racism in research beyond its implications for informed consent (Wolf 1999).

My interest in the Tuskegee Syphilis Study lies in what it can tell us about the adequacy of the existing standards, procedures, and practices that govern the use of human subjects in researching the differences between minorities and whites. I invoke Tuskegee not so much to identify contemporary research practices that might be considered abusive, but rather to call attention to features of the study that suggest how current research policies can be improved. Since being made public, the Tuskegee Syphilis Study has stood as a reminder of the need to protect vulnerable research subjects. I believe that the study may also offer valuable insights to guide the continued development of public policies and standards that seek to fairly distribute the benefits as well as the burdens of research through inclusion of members of disadvantaged and oppressed groups.

PERSONAL AND HISTORICAL COMMENTS

My personal interest in the Tuskegee Syphilis Study was triggered in 1972 when the story first broke. I was then serving as the deputy director of the Office of Civil Rights, U.S. Department of Health, Education, and Welfare (DHEW). In 1974, two years after the Tuskegee Syphilis Study came to light, Congress created the National Commission for the Protection of Human Subjects of Biomedical and Behavioral Research (National Commission). When I left the Office of Civil Rights in that same year, then–Secretary of Health, Education, and Welfare Caspar Weinberger, thinking that my civil rights experience would be relevant, asked if I would like to become a member of the fledgling National Commission. I accepted, and as a member, I analyzed the ramifications of the Tuskegee Syphilis Study in the development of the National Commission's *Belmont Report* (USDHEW 1979).

As a part of its work, the National Commission set out in its *Belmont Report* three principles to guide the conduct of research on human subjects—respect for persons, beneficence, and justice. The National Commission's formulation of the principle of justice emphasized distributive justice—that is, the fair allocation of research benefits and burdens. The National Commission was keenly aware of the disgraceful history of research abuses, both in the United States and abroad, and it specifically cited the Tuskegee Syphilis Study as an example of such an abuse. The National Commission's approach understandably reflected a desire to protect vulnerable subjects and "classes" of people, including African Americans, from undue burdens and risks. In the National Commission's view, important questions of individual and social justice are implicated when pools of subjects for human research studies are initially selected.

The view of the National Commission was that injustice or undue burden in research occurs when some classes are "systematically selected because of their easy availability, compromised position or their manipulability" (USDHEW 1979). To its credit, the National Commission embraced the view that not only individuals but, indeed, whole groups were at risk of exploitation in the research context (USDHEW 1979, 9). Regrettably, while the *Belmont Report* provides important guidance, it does not adequately explain how or why membership in a disadvantaged or oppressed group makes individual members of such groups particularly vulnerable (i.e., what was it about the subjects of the Tuskegee Syphilis Study and the context in which they lived that made them accessible?). Nor does the *Belmont Report* identify factors other than easy accessibility to describe why some groups and individuals are more vulnerable than others. The *Belmont Report* does note that injustice in the selection of subjects "arises from social, racial, sexual and cultural biases institutionalized in society" (USDHEW 1979, 19), yet the report does not explain how these factors impact research in ways that are potentially harmful to subjects. It should come as no surprise, therefore, that in the years following the issuance of the *Belmont Report*, minorities were excluded or underrepresented in research by the now-cautious scientific community.

In 1992, during the twentieth anniversary of the uncovering of the Tuskegee Syphilis Study, I was offered the opportunity to reflect on the significance of the study. In response to that request, I wrote what I think is my most influential, and surely most reproduced, article, "The Dangers of Difference" (King 1992). In that article, I stated that, although I understood that racial and ethnic minorities might benefit from increased attention to their health status, I was alarmed by the early efforts of the National Institutes of Health (NIH) to increase representation of women and minorities in clinical research pools.

In "The Dangers of Difference," I claimed that the Tuskegee Syphilis Study raised ethical and social issues for U.S. medicine's relationship with African Americans that were not broadly understood, appreciated, or even remembered. I warned that in a society riddled with racism and grounded in notions of white superiority, medical research into racial differences, while in some instances necessary, would likely be pursued in a manner that would ultimately burden rather than benefit African Americans. I believed that well-intentioned efforts to improve the health status of stigmatized groups might instead result in their harm.

In "The Dangers of Difference," I identified several perils involved in researching how, or indeed whether, race correlates to disease. First, the very idea of race is a confusing and ambiguous concept with doubtful biological (but not social) significance. Second, it is difficult to separate myth from reality when describing the relationship between race and disease, and the dangers posed by the myths of genetic differences and disease susceptibility are unmistakably illustrated by the United States' history with eugenics. Finally, research that calls attention to any disorders or conditions that occur disproportionately within a group might result in increased stigma and discrimination against the very group that the research sought to help.

The basis of my concerns included the NIH response to calls by women and minorities for greater inclusion in research populations. After the hiatus immediately following the issuance of *The Belmont Report*, a striking shift occurred in which the near-absolute exclusion of vulnerable subjects from studies gave way to the wide inclusion of woman and minorities in clinical research pools. This change was largely due to a shift in public perception in which clinical research came to be seen as potentially beneficial for the health status and health care of the individuals and groups studied rather than as merely a risky and burdensome venture. I worried that in moving from an era of protectionism in research to one of inclusion, new research policies which understandably focused on the prospect of benefit might not take sufficient account of their potential for harming vulnerable populations.

ADDRESSING UNDERREPRESENTATION IN CLINICAL RESEARCH

Calls for post–*Belmont Report* inclusion of African Americans into study populations first surfaced in the mid-1980s. In 1984, the U.S. Department of Health and Human Services (DHHS) established the Task Force on Black and Minority Health to examine health issues of blacks and other minorities, and the task force issued its report in 1985 (USDHHS 1985). The report called attention to the significant gaps that existed in scientific knowledge on the health status of African Americans and other minorities and noted the need for greater inclusion of racial and ethnic minorities in medical research. The report was largely ignored.

It was primarily the emergence of HIV/AIDS in the early 1980s that fostered the changing attitudes on the value of studying minority groups (Levine 1996, 105–26). HIV/AIDS grabbed public attention as a deadly syndrome that science was powerless to cure or control, and HIV/AIDS initially seemed to affect only one group in the United States—gay men, a group that was well-organized on health care issues. Gay activists saw inclusion in clinical research populations as being crucial to individual health and well-being, and they were prepared to challenge the assumptions of how research should be conducted. As the AIDS epidemic spread to other groups, including racial and ethnic minorities and other disadvantaged persons, the members of the newly affected subgroups also began to insist on access to research protocols. The formerly persuasive arguments for protecting minority groups from unethical treatment by excluding their members from research populations were suddenly outweighed by the interest in giving such persons their best hope for survival by granting access to the promising therapies available only in research trials (El-Sadr and Capps 1992).

In addition to the emerging view that members of minority groups combating particular illnesses should be allowed to participate in clinical trials of possible remedies, there grew a wider concern that women and minority health issues had been generally ignored. Some were concerned that too little attention had been paid to diseases and conditions that disproportionately affected minorities and women. In addition, some researchers questioned whether research results produced from trial groups that were overwhelmingly male and white were equally applicable to other groups (Dresser 1992).

The largely scientific question of whether research results obtained from populations that were overwhelmingly white and male were applicable to other population groups was not the only problem. This "one-size-fits-all" approach to research also implicitly established "white and male" as being equivalent to "normal." Such a practice labeled those other than white males as "different"—and, by implication, possibly inferior. Such assumptions were not only inappropriate in scientific protocols, they were also likely to reinforce culturally negative stereotypes of minority groups.

Continued pressure to include women and minorities as subjects in federally funded research culminated in the passage of the NIH Revitalization Act of 1993. The statute requires NIH to ensure that minorities and women are included in the study populations of all NIH-funded research. The original NIH Guidelines on the Inclusion of Women and Minorities as Subjects in Clinical Research (NIH 1994) implementing the legislation were amended in October 2001 (NIH 2001) to require investigators to categorize study participants into the racial and ethnic categories defined by Office of Management and Budget Directive No. 15. These groups are Hispanic or Latino, American Indian or Alaska Native, Asian, Black or African American, Native Hawaiian or other Pacific Islander, and White. Researchers must rely on the respondent's self-identification to collect data on race and ethnicity, and the respondent must be offered the opportunity to select more than one racial designation. Under these guidelines, research continues to consider the subjective criterion of race, notwithstanding the widespread consensus that race is not a strictly biological concept.

Laws and policies that seek to include underrepresented groups in research pools are supported by the ethical principles of beneficence and justice as developed in *The Belmont Report* (Weijer 1996). However, a necessary side effect of such inclusion policies is that, in striving to account for and protect the interests of specific subgroups, researchers must focus great attention on the physical differences of the groups studied. This focus might be beneficial—as, for example, when uncovering disparities in health. Lurking within this style of research, however, is also the possibility that research data collected from different racially representative research pools might identify significant genetic differences among the subgroups studied. These possibilities raise a dilemma.

On the one hand, if real biological differences are identified between minority research groups and the white male "norm," then it is reasonable to assume that past research strategies may have benefited the health status of white males to the detriment of other groups (Bovet and Paccaud 2001) and that affirmative efforts to rectify the knowledge gap are warranted. Furthermore, if specific health problems are discovered to be linked to specific minority subgroups, difficult issues of research priorities are implicated. Fair distribution of research burdens and benefits would seem to require examination of potentially discriminatory policies and practices well beyond those that could be solved by the mere increase of representation in clinical trials. Therefore, racial and ethnic minorities potentially benefit from research that targets the diseases and conditions that disproportionately affect them.

On the other hand, the prospect of identifying significant health disparities or biological differences in minority racial or ethnic groups carries with it the possibility of feeding existing negative stereotypes, biases, and racist ideologies. The possible existence of non–sex-trait genetic differences between men and women is relatively uncontroversial (Levine 1991; Dresser 1992), but the possibility of discovering significant genetic differences between racial and ethnic minorities on one side and whites on the other is another matter entirely. In the past, belief in such differences supported practices that were harmful.

At the time that adoption of inclusion policies was being considered, it was reasonable to believe that important biological differences between racial subgroups might be uncovered. For example, it was widely known that sickle-cell anemia, a genetic disease, disproportionately affected persons of African descent, and there was evidence in the research literature to support the existence of differential responses to pharmacological interventions. Indeed, James E. Bowman and Robert Murray, distinguished African American physicians and academicians, described the prospect of such biological differences in their book *Genetic Variation and Disorders in Peoples of African Origin* (Bowman and Murray 1990).

However, few called attention either to the likelihood of uncovering genetic differences or to the risks that such discoveries might raise. It is reasonable to speculate that the reason for the silence on this issue was a fear of possibly undermining the gains made by the civil rights movement and its emphasis on cross-racial similarities. After all, it had only been since passage of the Civil Rights Act of 1964 that discrimination in health care institutions receiving federal funds had been prohibited (Smedley, Stith, and Nelson 2002). Ultimately, the roles of race and ethnicity were downplayed, and inclusionary policies were adopted without adequate consideration of the potential risks they posed to various minority groups—especially African Americans.[2]

TUSKEGEE'S LESSONS

In the past decade, minority health concerns have received a great deal of attention. In 1990, the NIH Office of Research on Minority Health was created, and in 1998, President William Jefferson Clinton announced the goal of eliminating racial and ethnic disparities in U.S. health care by the year 2010. In 2002, the National Academy of Science's Institute of Medicine completed a major study of racial and ethnic disparities in U.S. health care (Smedley, Stith, and Nelson 2002). Racial identification has been a necessary element in the federal government's attempts to identify the social and economic influences that contribute to racial and ethnic disparities in health, and such identification has clearly played an important role in promoting fair and beneficial public policies for racial and ethnic minorities. However, while there has been much progress in the past ten years, the problems identified in my 1992 article still exist, and the rise of the genetic era of medicine is likely to exacerbate them. Although I believe that important lessons from the Tuskegee Syphilis Study were largely overlooked by policymakers at the time inclusionary policies were adopted, it is not too late to consider their relevance for contemporary controversies that flow from these policies.

The Tuskegee study demonstrates the many ways in which individuals and groups can be put at risk by participation in medical research. As noted above, the Tuskegee study is useful in understanding why the members of easily accessible groups are at risk for coercion and exploitation in research. The study was conducted in the rural, poor, and segregated Deep South. The subjects' lack of economic resources limited their access to health care and made them vulnerable to the promise of free medical care.

The African American males who were chosen as subjects of the Tuskegee Syphilis Study were isolated geographically and psychologically from both whites and middle-class African Americans, and as the study began in the midst of the Depression, the subjects were politically powerless in a profound way. The prevailing culture of their time devalued them as human beings, and the reason for their easy accessibility simply cannot be understood without acknowledging the racism that dominated the culture in which they lived. Later, when penicillin, though available, was not provided to the subjects, a factor that surely contributed to that decision was the perception that the lives of the subjects (and the lives of their spouses and children) were not valuable.

In contemporary society, where so many minorities lack health insurance and so many others receive health coverage or care from public programs, minority communities continue to be fertile grounds for recruiting subjects. The possibility of receiving an individual benefit in a free clinical trial might be more alluring to minorities than whites, and minorities are accordingly disproportionately vulnerable to the associated risk of physical harms and to the risk of being taken advantage of as a group.

The Tuskegee Syphilis Study also serves to remind us of society's obsession with differences between human beings and of society's tendency to favor biological over social, economic, and cultural explanations of these differences. Significantly, "the Tuskegee Study's design itself was predicated on an epidemiological finding: the wide disparity in patterns of disease between African Americans and whites" (Brandt and Churchill 2000, xv–xvi). The Tuskegee Syphilis Study was designed to investigate the effects of untreated syphilis only on the Negro male, as a study of untreated syphilis in whites had already been conducted in Oslo, Norway, by Dr. E. Bruusgaard (Jones 1993, 92–93). The Tuskegee researchers selected blacks for their study because, in keeping with the science of the day, they believed that the course of syphilis in blacks might differ from what had been observed in whites. When reviewing an early outline of the study, Dr. Joseph Earle Moore of the Venereal Disease Clinic of the Johns Hopkins University School of Medicine went so far as to opine that "syphilis in the Negro is in many respects almost a different disease from syphilis in the white" (Jones 1993, 106). Specifically, it was thought that the disease was more likely to attack the neural system in whites and the cardiovascular system in blacks. This belief is curious, since even at the time there was little evidence to support it, and test subjects of different races were, in fact, given the same treatment for the disease (Jones 1993, 106).

Dr. Raymond Vonderlehr, a researcher at the USPHS appointed to head the Tuskegee Syphilis Study, was particularly interested in cardiovascular syphilis. During physical examinations of prospective subjects, Vonderlehr X-rayed the syphilitic applicants and uncovered so many cases of cardiovascular involvement that other researchers were consulted to verify his findings. Upon reviewing the X-ray readings, Dr. Joseph E. Moore concluded: "Doctor Von der Lehr seems to have uncovered a perfect gold mine of cardiovascular syphilis" (Jones 1993, 122). Later, however, Dr. Vonderlehr sought confirmation of his findings from the American Heart Association. According to Jones:

> The response was devastating. Dr. Vonderlehr's most important finding to date had been a high incidence of cardiovascular syphilis, and he had turned to the American Heart Association hoping to have his diagnoses confirmed. Instead, the spokesman for the organization, Dr. H. M. Marvin, totally rejected the scientific validity of the procedures and tests upon which the diagnoses had been based. Dr. Marvin's conclusions were supported by a blue ribbon panel composed of specialists. Dr. Marvin believed that the diagnoses were hopelessly subjective observations. (Jones 1993, 139)

Despite the prestige and authority of the American Heart Association, the report did not change Vonderlehr's views of his diagnoses. He dismissed the matter as a mere difference of opinion.

This episode reminds us that researchers are not immune to the prevailing perceptions of the cultures in which they live and work. The Tuskegee researchers believed that blacks and whites had different diseases and would not seek treatment for syphilis or other diseases. They believed that blacks were promiscuous and of a different sexual nature than whites. These medical professionals participated in a culture in which "social Darwinists," armed with a new rationale for racism, asserted that the Negro could not win the struggle to survive (Brandt 2000). Moreover, it was the medical profession that provided much of the data that was used to support innate racial differences (Jones 1993). These prevailing attitudes and negative stereotypes about blacks played an important role in shaping the design and implementation of the Tuskegee study.

Scientific research in the twenty-first century is not immune from similar forces. A recent report of the Institute of Medicine makes a critical finding:

Finding 4-1: Bias, stereotyping, prejudice, and clinical uncertainty on the part of health care providers may contribute to racial and ethnic disparities in health care. While indirect evidence from several lines of research supports this statement, a greater understanding of the prevalence and influence of these processes is needed and should be sought through research. (Smedley, Stith, and Nelson 2002)

The Tuskegee Syphilis Study, however, does more than just remind us of our fascination with differences. The Tuskegee study prompts us to recall the reasons for medicine's absorption with demonstrating physical and mental differences between blacks and whites. Scientific evidence that demonstrated differences could also justify white superiority. As James Jones points out:

Most physicians . . . who wrote about blacks during the nineteenth century believed in the social order. They justified slavery and, after its abolition, second-class citizenship by insisting that blacks were incapable of assuming any higher station in life. Too many differences separated the races. And here "different" unquestionably meant "inferior." (Jones 1993, 17)

The essential message of Tuskegee is that while emphasizing differences in medicine can lead to favorable treatment, it can just as easily support differential and abusive treatment of others. Consequently, it is critical that suspected biological differences between population groups be subjected to the most careful and rigorous scrutiny before they become the basis of scientific studies.

One of the consequences of adopting inclusionary policies in clinical research is that clinical investigations identifying differential responses between blacks and whites are being conducted with ever-greater frequency. Race is still prioritized as a relevant biological factor, notwithstanding its dubious scientific value (Osborne and Feit 1992).

The results of the Human Genome Project (the program to map and sequence the human genome) have complicated rather than simplified the task of understanding the biological significance of race. This is so because at the same time that the Human Genome Project demonstrates that race is irrelevant, its results are used to identify genetic variation among racial subgroups. This apparent incongruity understandably confuses many.

On the one hand, information from the Human Genome Project supports the conclusion that there is no biological basis for race in humans. Humans are 99.9 percent alike, and while there is normal genetic diversity among humans, this variation is overwhelmingly at the individual level, rather than the population level (Collins 2001). In short, there is far too little variation among so-called racial subgroups of humans to support the idea that these subgroups are distinct evolutionary lineages.

However, medicine is rightly interested in exploring human differences at the molecular level that may lead to more effective interventions, and the frequency of genes that might play a role in predisposition to disease or to drug response does vary among population groups. The critical question, however, is whether any identified genetic variation for disease incidence or drug response is coextensive with *socially* defined categories of race and ethnicity (Graves 2001, 173–92). It is entirely possible that a person labeled "white" might be more genetically similar to someone labeled "Native American" than to another white. Can (and should) important differences among humans be identified by reliance on socially constructed categories of race and ethnicity?

Controversy about these concerns exploded into public view in the May 2001 issue of the *New England Journal of Medicine* (NEJM). The controversy reveals the extent to which inclusion policies that seek to identify differences between blacks and whites, while potentially beneficial, are still in need of attention from policymakers in order to prevent unintended harms. In that issue of NEJM, the results of two studies relevant to the question were published. One study concluded that administering enalapril, an angiotensin-converting-enzyme (ACE) inhibitor, was associated with a significant reduction in the risk of hospitalization for heart failure among white patients with left ventricular dysfunction, but not among black patients (Exner et al. 2001). The second study concluded that carvedilol, a beta-blocker, was of equal benefit to both black and non-black patients with chronic heart disease (Yancy et al. 2001).

These important studies were accompanied by two editorials. The first, written by Robert S. Schwartz, M.D., a deputy editor of NEJM, argued that the authors of the studies "refer to 'race,' 'racial groups,' 'racial differences,' and 'ethnic background' but offer no plausible biological explanation for making such distinctions" (Schwartz 2001, 1392). Schwartz's point is that "attributing differences in a biologic end point to race is not only imprecise but also of no proven value in treating an individual patient" (Schwartz 2001, 1392). The other editorial, written by Alastair J. J. Wood, M.D., argues that the two articles "address the effect of race on the response to drugs of two important classes used in heart failure . . . [and] will . . . be of great help to physicians in their attempt to choose the best therapy for heart failure in patients of different races" (Wood 2001, 1394).

The editorialists seem to agree that individually tailored interventions are the ultimate goal of important pharmaceutical research. Schwartz argues that racial designations have no place in clinical medicine or re-search, stating that "publication of the first draft of the human genome should force an end to medical research that is arbitrarily based on race" (Schwartz 2001, 1392). Wood points out that the impact of racial differ-ences on response to drug interventions "should alert physicians to the important underlying genetic determinants of drug response," and that the next step "will be the identification of genetic determinants of the reported racial differences, rather than attention to the external manifesta-tions of race" (Wood 2001, 1395). Wood understands that membership in a socially defined racial group is a poor proxy for the full panoply of individual human genetic variation, but he thinks that it offers important information that can be of immediate practical clinical use. He anticipates the need for additional studies that go beyond race, but he does not offer suggestions about how such studies should be structured. Schwartz believes that researchers and journals should take measures now to mini-mize the use of race as a variable in research.

What policies should be adopted to "move beyond race" or guide a transition? Tuskegee's lessons have application here. A critical first step would be to devise a research program that would explore many plausible explanations for the differences that have been detected. Differences between blacks and whites in disease susceptibilities and responses to clinical interventions may be the result of genetic differences, environmental factors (including shared cultural and dietary differences), or fundamental differences in the pathogenesis of diseases. All of the possible contributors—not just genetics—should be examined.

If biological differences are detected, should there be continued reliance on skin color and other phenotypic manifestations, which are of dubious validity? Should the next clinical trial of, for example, enalapril enroll only white subjects because they alone appear to benefit from the intervention? The Food and Drug Administration recently approved the first clinical trial of a drug designed for African Americans only—BiDil. The trial, which will enroll only African American test subjects, is sponsored by NitroMed, Inc., and the Association of Black Cardiologists. It is not immediately clear why the study should be conducted in this race-attentive manner. Wouldn't it be preferable to involve both black and white test subjects, so that specific causal factors could be identified by comparing subjects of both groups who responded favorably, or unfavorably, to the drug? After all, as described above, differences in skin color can mask genetic similarities, while similarity in skin color can mask genetic differences.

A worrisome prospect is that generalized differences in racial responses to drugs may become a basis for diagnosis and therapy. In response to the two studies discussed above, some physicians no longer prescribe ACE inhibitors for the treatment of heart disease in blacks (Masoudi and Havranek 2001). If a future clinical trial enrolling only blacks or whites is established, the likelihood of affecting diagnostic and therapeutic practices is even greater. This development is alarming because the continued use of socially defined race as an indicator in making scientific prescription choices could lead to both white and black patients receiving substandard care (some blacks will receive drugs that they should not, while some whites will be denied a drug which might benefit them). Nonetheless, Wood and other physicians genuinely concerned with helping their patients but facing medical uncertainties in diagnosing and treating them would argue that stereotyping patients by race provides a clue as to which therapy is most appropriate, and a clue, any clue, is better than nothing (Satel 2002).

Adoption of research policies in a transition to individually tailored therapies requires making difficult trade-offs between potentially short-term benefits and long-term burdens. The events at Tuskegee caution that research should be designed and conducted in a way that does not reinforce the perception of white superiority. When only African Americans (as opposed to only whites) are used as test subjects in a clinical trial, this surely opens up the possibility of future stigma and discrimination. One can envision a future where drugs only known to benefit persons of African descent are not developed for fear that they will be too expensive for black patients to afford, or where African Americans are labeled genetically inferior because their response to a particular drug is different from that of whites or other groups.

There are, of course, no easy answers to the question of how medicine should make the transition away from using race-based research to identify genetic and other causes of disease. The Tuskegee Syphilis Study warns that including minorities in clinical research might improve the well-being of individuals and groups but only if there is attention to the context in which the research takes place. Research that produces ambiguous or ill-defined correlations between race and disease risks rekindling debates over the relative roles of heredity versus environment, and the negative impact of renewing arguments over genetically superior versus genetically inferior groups of humans might overwhelm any potential positive impact on minority health status.

Some practices can be modified relatively quickly. Researchers should take pains to accurately describe their results when they submit their articles for publication. They might, for example, be required by journals in which they publish to describe their study populations with relevant scientific terms rather than simply using categories such as "black" or "African American" and "white"—terms that perpetuate misperceptions while contributing little (Bhopal and Donaldson 1998). Indeed, the development of a "standard lexicon" of accurate, neutral, and nonstigmatizing language should be a priority of funding agencies (Rothenberg and Rutkin 1998).

There are, of course, no easy answers to the question of how medicine should make the transition away from using race-based research to identify genetic and other causes of disease. However, I believe that the Tuskegee Syphilis Study offers lessons that we should heed when considering this matter, as it demonstrates the many ways in which minorities can be put at risk in medical research. Only when we fully recognize the potential pitfalls of race-based research can we design policies and protocols that can benefit minority groups without harming them.

NOTES

1. I use the term "subject" rather than "participant" because I agree with Commissioner Alexander Morgan Capron and others who observe that "*[p]articipant* might be a fine term of aspiration, but it is premature to adopt the term, because too many patients and volunteers who are enrolled in research studies are still not free and equal participants in the research; indeed, changing the term could send a false signal that less vigilance is needed to protect human subjects . . ." (National Bioethics Advisory Commission 2001, 33).

2. Although I frequently use the term "minorities," my focus is African Americans. Women and other racial and ethnic minorities have separate and distinct experiences with American medicine. See, for example, Mastroianni, Faden, and Federman 1994.

REFERENCES

Bhopal, Raj, and Liam Donaldson. 1998. White, European, Western, Caucasian, or What? Inappropriate Labeling in Research on Race, Ethnicity, and Health. *American Journal of Public Health* 88: 1303–7.

Bovet, Pascal, and Fred Paccaud. 2001. Letter to the editor. *The New England Journal of Medicine* 345: 767.

Bowman, James E., and Robert Murray. 1990. *Genetic Variation and Disorders in Peoples of African Origin*. Baltimore: Johns Hopkins University Press.

Brandt, Allan. 2000. Racism and Research: The Case of the Tuskegee Syphilis Experiment. In *Tuskegee's Truths*, edited by Susan Reverby. Chapel Hill: University of North Carolina Press.

Brandt, Allan M., and Larry R. Churchill. 2000. Preface. In *Tuskegee's Truths*, edited by Susan Reverby. Chapel Hill: University of North Carolina Press.

Byrd, W., and Linda Clayton. 2000. *An American Health Dilemma*. Vol. 1. New York: Routledge.

Collins, Francis S. 2001. *Testimony of Francis S. Collins, M.D., Ph.D., Director, National Human Genome Research Institute, National Institutes of Health, Before the Health, Education, Labor, and Pensions Committee, United States Senate*. www.genome.gov/page.cfm?page ID=10003482 (visited July 13, 2002).

Dresser, Rebecca. 1992. Wanted: Single, White Male for Medical Research. *Hastings Center Report* 22: 24–29.

El-Sadr, Walfaa, and Linnea Capps. 1992. The Challenge of Minority Recruitment in Clinical Trials for AIDS. *Journal of the American Medical Association* 267: 954–57.

Exner, Derek, Daniel L. Drier, Michael J. Domanski, and Jay N. Cohn. 2001. Lesser Response to Angiotensin-Converting-Enzyme Inhibitor Therapy in Black as Compared with White Patients with Left Ventricular Dysfunction. *The New England Journal of Medicine* 344: 1351–57.

Graves, Joseph L. 2001. *The Emperor's New Clothes: Biological Theories of Race at the End of the Millennium.* New Brunswick, N.J.: Rutgers University Press.

Jones, James H. 1993. *Bad Blood: The Tuskegee Syphilis Experiment.* New York: Free Press.

King, Patricia A. 1992. The Dangers of Difference. *Hastings Center Report* 22: 35–38.

Levine, Carol. 1991. Women and HIV/AIDS Research: The Barriers to Equity. *IRB: A Review of Human Subjects Research* 13(1–2): 1–6.

———. 1996. Changing Views of Justice after Belmont: AIDS and the Inclusion of Vulnerable Subjects. In *The Ethics of Research Involving Human Subjects: Facing the Twenty-first Century*, edited by Harold Y. Vanderpool. Frederick, Md.: University Publishing Group, 105–26.

Masoudi, Frederick, and Edward P. Havranek. 2001. Letter to the editor. *The New England Journal of Medicine* 345: 767.

Mastroianni, Anna C., Ruth Faden, and Daniel Federman 1994. *Women and Health Research: Ethical and Legal Issues of Including Women in Research.* Vol. 1. Washington, D.C.: National Academy Press.

National Bioethics Advisory Commission. 2001. *Ethical and Policy Issues in Research Involving Human Participants.* Vol. 1. Bethesda, Md.: National Bioethics Advisory Commission.

National Institutes of Health. 1994. *NIH Guidelines on the Inclusion of Women and Minorities as Subjects in Clinical Research. March 1994.* http://grants.nih.gov/grants/guide/notice-files/not94-100.html (visited July 13, 2002).

———. 2001. *NIH Policy and Guidelines on the Inclusion of Women and Minorities as Subjects in Clinical Research—Amended October 2001.* http://grants2.nih.gov/grants/funding/women_min/guidelines_amended_10_2001.htm (visited July 13, 2002).

NIH Revitalization Act of 1993. PL 103-43; Public Health Service Act. 1994. U.S. Code. Vol. 42, sec. 289a-2.

Osborne, Newton G., and Marvin D. Feit. 1992. The Use of Race in Medical Research. *Journal of the American Medical Association* 267, no. 2 (January 8, 1992).

Reverby, Susan. 2000. *Tuskegee's Truths: Rethinking the Tuskegee Syphilis Study.* Chapel Hill: University of North Carolina Press.

Rothenberg, Karen H., and Amy B. Rutkin, 1998. Toward a Framework of Mutualism: The Jewish Community in Genetics Research. *Community Genetics* 1: 148–53.

Satel, Sally. 2002. I Am a Racially Profiling Doctor. *New York Times Magazine*, May 5, 2002, sec. 6.

Schwartz, R. S. 2001. Racial Profiling in Medical Research. *The New England Journal of Medicine* 344: 1392.

Smedley, Brian D., Adrienne Y. Stith, and Alan R. Nelson. 2002. *Unequal Treatment: Confronting Racial and Ethnic Disparities in Health Care.* Washington, D.C.: National Academy Press.

U.S. Department of Health and Human Services (USDHHS). Task Force on Black and Minority Health. 1985. *Report of the Secretary's Task Force on Black and Minority Health.* Vol. I. Washington, D.C.: Government Printing Office.

U.S. Department of Health, Education, and Welfare, National Commission for the Protection of Human Subjects of Biomedical and Behavioral Research. 1979. *Ethical Principles and Guidelines for the Protection of Human Subjects of Research (Belmont Report).* Washington, D.C.: Government Printing Office.

Weijer, Charles. 1996. Evolving Ethical Issues in Selection of Subjects for Clinical Research. *Cambridge Quarterly of Healthcare Ethics* 5: 334–45.

Wolf, Susan. 1999. Erasing Difference: Race, Ethnicity, and Gender in Bioethics. In *Embodying Bioethics*, edited by Anne Donchin and Laura Purdy. Lanham, Md.: Rowman & Littlefield.

Wood, A. J. J. 2001. Racial Differences in the Response to Drugs: Pointers to Genetic Differences. *The New England Journal of Medicine* 344: 1393–95.

Yancy, C. W., et al. 2001. Race and the Response to Adrenergic Blockade with Carvedilol in Patients with Chronic Heart Failure. *The New England Journal of Medicine* 344: 1358–65.

The Birth and Youth of the Kennedy Institute of Ethics

LeROY WALTERS

I would like to explore some of the factors that contributed to the establishment, the development, and—if it is not too immodest to talk this way—the success of the Kennedy Institute during its first thirty years. This exploration will inevitably be an interpretation of the Institute's thirty-year history. Because of space constraints, it will also be highly selective.

The Institute would not be here were it not for the vision of André Hellegers and Sargent and Eunice Kennedy Shriver. Thus, I would like to begin by acknowledging a debt to these three creative and thoughtful people.

A first characteristic of the Kennedy Institute, from the time of its inception, was its *international* focus. André Hellegers himself was a citizen of the world. He had been born in the Netherlands and educated in England, Scotland, and France before moving to the United States as his new home in 1953. While living in the United States, André maintained close ties with the rest of the world, and especially with his native Europe. In the 1960s, before most of us had ever met him, he served as deputy director to the Papal Commission on Birth Control. He thoroughly enjoyed interacting with this international group of scholars, which sought to review and perhaps to revise the Catholic Church's traditional teaching on contraception. I remember his frequent trips to Europe and his desire to stay in touch with intellectual and ecclesiastical developments there during the 1970s. Not long before his death André compiled a summary of recent developments in bioethics for the Vatican, totally on his own. He was constantly aware of the global character of his church and of the questions that faced the then-just-emerging field of bioethics.

Since the 1960s, the Shrivers have also had a keen interest in the international dimensions of bioethics. Already in 1967, the Kennedy Foundation and Harvard Divinity School had cosponsored an international conference on abortion, to which both European and North

American scholars were invited. In October 1971, within months of the Kennedy Institute's opening, the Foundation sponsored an international conference with the theme "Choices on Our Conscience." Speakers from Europe joined their North American colleagues in exploring some of the major issues of that time.

It should thus be no surprise that the Kennedy Institute itself has always sought to be global in its outlook. This international character of the Institute has expressed itself in many ways. Our visiting scholars have come from every corner of the globe. During the summer of 1979, Institute faculty members joined Sargent Shriver and John Collins Harvey to explore new territory—bioethics in China and Japan. Our long-term colleagues, Rihito Kimura from Japan and Hans-Martin Sass from Germany, have reminded us that other cultures and philosophical and religious traditions may view the world and biomedical technology in a way that differs from, say, Anglo-American philosophy and theology. When Warren Reich and his associate editors planned the first edition of the *Encyclopedia of Bioethics* (Reich 1978), they made it a decisively international compendium of knowledge.

Under Doris Goldstein's leadership, the Bioethics Library has also been international in its coverage, constrained only by our limited knowledge of non-Western languages. Bioethics scholars from around the world view the library as their information mecca and make as many pilgrimages to this academic shrine as their time and budgets will allow. While the bioethics information retrieval project limits itself to English-language materials, our librarians and bibliographers scan the world in their search for bioethics literature. And Bob Veatch teaches an entire course on cross-cultural approaches to bioethics.

The two seminal works in bioethics that perhaps best illustrate the international focus of the Institute are the previously mentioned *Encyclopedia of Bioethics* and the annual *Bibliography of Bioethics.* In the first edition of the *Encyclopedia*, published in 1978, an international group of authors produced surveys of medical ethics in the following societies, regions, and nations: primitive societies, the ancient Near East, ancient Greece and Rome, sub-Saharan Africa, Latin America, Israel, Persia, the Arab world, India, Japan, China, Britain, France, Central Europe, Eastern Europe, and North America. The approximately thirty *Encyclopedia* articles devoted to this international review provide an informative overview of bioethics-related questions that have been discussed in diverse cultures and regions of our world. This global perspective is enhanced and updated by thirty-four similar articles included in the second edition of the *Encyclopedia*, published in 1995 (Reich 1995).

The *Bibliography of Bioethics* is a second reference work that illustrates the Kennedy Institute's strong international focus (Walters and Kahn 2002). Initially published in 1975, the *Bibliography* has always sought to include English-language materials published anywhere in the world. Most bioethics-related documents published in Canada, the United Kingdom, Australia, New Zealand, and the United States were initially written in English and thus were immediately captured by the bioethics information retrieval system that underlies the *Bibliography*. In addition, just as English is increasingly becoming the primary language for publications in science and medicine, it has gradually emerged as the most important language for international bioethics. Thus, bioethics scholars in Europe, Asia, Africa, and Latin America regularly publish their work in English.

There is a second way in which the *Bibliography* has contributed to global bioethics research. The Bioethics Thesaurus was initially developed in 1974 and 1975 as a small, cross-disciplinary set of terms to be used in indexing documents for the annual *Bibliography*. From an initial size of 500 terms, the thesaurus gradually expanded to its current size of approximately 700 terms (not including proper names). Since its creation, the Bioethics Thesaurus has been translated into Spanish, French, German, Dutch, and Swedish; it is currently being translated into Turkish. The information scientists and documentation experts who have translated the thesaurus have, of course, revised it and added concepts that are important in their languages but less important (or even absent) in English. Nonetheless, the Bioethics Thesaurus has helped to facilitate an international standardization in the way that bioethics documents are indexed in multiple languages and cultures.

A second characteristic of the Kennedy Institute that has been present from the beginning is its *interdisciplinary* character. Again in this case, André Hellegers's experience with the Papal Commission was undoubtedly a formative influence. André delighted in the fruitful interchange that he experienced among natural scientists (biologists and physicians), social scientists (especially demographers), and humanities scholars (especially theologians). While at Johns Hopkins University in the 1960s, André sought to promote similar interdisciplinary dialogue, but the effort never really took off. He thus sought a new venue, a Jesuit university, with a much less prestigious medical school but perhaps a greater openness, across multiple campuses, to such interdisciplinary work.

The Shrivers and André Hellegers collaborated in promoting interdisci-plinary approaches in several ways. The 1967 conference on abortion and the 1971 symposium "Choices on Our Conscience" included scholars and public intellectuals from multiple backgrounds and academic fields. Less obvious, but equally important in my view, is the way that the Kennedy Foundation and André made it possible for Paul Ramsey to do pioneering interdisciplinary work. During the spring semesters of 1968 and 1969, the Shrivers and André arranged for Paul to immerse himself in conversations with clinicians and biomedical researchers at Georgetown University and the National Institutes of Health (NIH), to attend case conferences and rounds, and to devour a tremendous quantity of biomedi-cal literature. One of Paul Ramsey's most impressive achievements in *The Patient as Person* (Ramsey 1970a) was to draw upon and synthesize the literature of biology and medicine, law, theology, and the daily newspaper. In fact, one could create an excellent bibliography of bioethics through late 1969 simply by arranging the bibliographic references in Paul's footnotes under ten or twelve major topics. In my view, Paul's success in bridging the disciplines was one of the major factors that convinced the Kennedy Foundation to fund a high-risk venture—the establishment of a research institute for human reproduction and bioethics.

Through a quirk of history, the Kennedy Institute began as a collabora-tion among a physician, a small group of theologians, and a small group of demographers. However, the turn toward the inclusion of other disciplines occurred early and often. In 1974 Leon Kass, who held an M.D. degree and a Ph.D. in biochemistry, joined the Institute. During the same year, Seymour Perlin, a psychiatrist, became a visiting scholar. Our law school colleagues, Patricia King and Judith Areen, became increasingly interested in bioethics. Tom Beauchamp, influenced by a 1974 summer workshop on bioethics led by Samuel Gorovitz, began to collaborate with several of our Institute colleagues, especially Jim Childress, and made the first strong philosophical contribution to the life of the Institute. Then, through the generosity of the Kennedy Foundation, philosopher Tris Engelhardt (who also had an M.D. degree) became a long-term member of the Kennedy Institute. At about the same time, we were joined on a part-time basis by Ruth Faden, who held a Ph.D. in psychology and brought her more empirical approach to the Institute and the field of bioethics. In two stints as a visiting scholar, historian James Jones wrote the definitive account of the Tuskegee Syphilis Study. In 1983, Edmund Pellegrino, a distinguished physician, became director of the Institute. And thirteen years ago our first lawyer and philosopher, Madison Powers, joined us as a faculty colleague. I regret that time does not permit me to acknowledge individually the tremendous contributions that theologians Roy Branson, Bill May, Bob Veatch, and Bryan Hehir; philosophers John Langan, Maggie Little, and Kevin Wildes; physician-theologian John Collins Harvey; physician-philosopher Dan Sulmasy; and nurse-philosopher Carol Taylor have also made to the intellectual life of the Institute.

In the early years of the Kennedy Institute there was not always a perfect fit between demography and bioethics, and the involvement of our biomedical colleagues, except for Leon Kass, Bob Baumiller, Francesc Abel, and André, was always sporadic. However, the ideal of being interdisciplinary in our approach was always firmly fixed in our minds. The *Encyclopedia of Bioethics*, published in 1978, was a monumental work of interdisciplinarity. As our librarians gathered literature for the Bioethics Library, they did not care what disciplinary label had been applied to a book or an article. If the document was relevant to the field of bioethics, it was added to the collection and became a candidate for inclusion in the *Bibliography of Bioethics*. The course syllabi of Institute faculty members also defy traditional disciplinary boundaries.

I will briefly mention two vignettes to illustrate the payoff of the Institute's interdisciplinary approach. When I was invited to comment on the draft NIH guidelines for recombinant DNA research in early 1976, I remember going to Leon Kass to ask for suggestions about what books to read. Leon pointed me in the direction of *The Molecular Biology of the Gene* by James Watson and others. Leon was also very tolerant of my ignorance about basic biology. When I asked him what the difference between a bacterial virus and a bacteriophage was, he did not laugh me out of court but patiently explained that these were two terms for the same entity.

A second vignette also remains vivid in my memory. André Hellegers had a weakness for saying yes to invitations from community and religious groups wanting to learn "something about bioethics." Often he would invite some of us to join him. I remember one occasion on which André, Judith Areen, Tom Beauchamp, and I journeyed to a Catholic parish in northern Virginia. The small audience that evening was treated to an interdisciplinary panel comprised of a physician, a lawyer, a philosopher, and a person trained in theology. As the discussion unfolded, it became clear that the four of us did not agree on the ethical and legal issues surrounding abortion. André was pleased that we had demonstrated the value of an interdisciplinary approach and that we had stimulated the thinking of our audience through presenting multiple points of view.

It is an open secret that André had a favorite among the disciplines that he hoped would contribute to the field of bioethics. That discipline was *theology*. Think for a moment about his early collaboration with Paul Ramsey. Note also that most of the early visiting scholars to the Institute and the first two long-term faculty members were moral theologians. In 1973, the Shrivers and André agreed that the two endowed chairs to be created at the Institute would be called chairs in *Christian ethics*—thus making it likely that most future holders of those chairs would be theologically trained. The soft spot in André's heart for theologians will be obvious to anyone who studies the early history of the Kennedy Institute. What is less well known is how vigorously he tried to promote theological scholarship at Georgetown, in general. When the news broke in 1973 that the Woodstock Theological Seminary would shortly close, Yale University and Union Theological Seminary in New York made strong bids for the venerable Woodstock Library. In André's view, the only appropriate location for this priceless collection was Georgetown University. With the assent of Georgetown's president, Robert Henle, André orchestrated a massive letter-writing campaign, urging the decision makers in the Society of Jesus to award this prize to Georgetown. His campaign succeeded. In 1974 the collection moved to Georgetown, and André was able to celebrate the library's opening on the Georgetown campus in the fall of 1975. All of us are indebted to André for the special affection that he showed toward theology and toward the books and journals that support research in this field.

A seminal work that vividly illustrates the Institute's interdisciplinary character was in fact published a year before the Institute was established. It is the aforementioned book *The Patient as Person*, written by Paul Ramsey in 1968 and 1969 and published in 1970 by Yale University Press (Ramsey 1970a). Before meeting the Shrivers and André, Paul, a Yale-trained Methodist moral theologian, had twice written essays on bioethical themes. In a 1956 symposium published by New York University's law school, Paul had responded to Joseph Fletcher's 1954 book *Morals and Medicine* in an essay titled "Freedom and Responsibility in Medical and Sex Ethics: A Protestant View" (Ramsey 1956). Similarly, in a 1965 paper presented during a symposium held at Gustavus Adolphus College, Paul had launched a frontal assault on positive eugenics under the title "Moral and Religious Implications of Genetic Control" (Ramsey 1966).[1] However, neither of these earlier essays presaged the kind of creative interdisciplinary synthesis that Paul was able to achieve in *The Patient as Person*.

What was the genius of this 1970 book? First, Paul identified a major theological theme, loyalty to covenantal commitments, and translated it both into Kantian philosophical terms (an ethic of means) and into a set of fiduciary duties that health professionals and researchers owed to patients and research subjects. In Paul's view, the consent of a patient or subject was not a legalistic requirement—and especially not a matter of signing a document. Rather, consent was a "canon of loyalty" between the powerful professional and the relatively vulnerable patient or subject (Ramsey 1970a, 2).

Second, in *The Patient as Person* Paul promoted interdisciplinary discussion by avoiding topics that were identified with theological (and especially Catholic) medical ethics. In this book there are no discussions of contraception, abortion, prenatal diagnosis, or assisted reproduction. Instead, the book deals with major themes that continue to be central to bioethics and to cultural debates in all industrialized nations. What are the moral obligations of researchers to research subjects—and especially to children, to people with intellectual disabilities, and to institutionalized people? What does it mean to care for a dying person, and what are various forms that care might take? How can we ensure that gravely ill patients will not prematurely be declared dead because of our desire to transplant their still-living organs into other patients? And how can scarce resources like (at that time) renal dialysis be allocated to candidates in a way that shows respect for every human being and avoids invidious judgments about comparative social worth?

Finally, as noted earlier, Paul's book promoted interdisciplinary discussion by being well documented and thoroughly up-to-date on the debates that were actually occurring in the literature of medicine, law, theology, and government documents, as well as in the popular press. Even though the Willowbrook studies of hepatitis in institutionalized children had been conducted in the 1950s, they were a matter for ongoing discussion in at least one major medical journal. The story of the Seattle selection committee, which had made life-and-death decisions about candidates for renal dialysis, had been brought to public attention by a thoughtful journalist, Shana Alexander, and published in *Life* magazine. Paul's voracious reading and his ongoing conversations with biomedical experts like George Schreiner in nephrology and Leon Kass in medicine more generally made him a credible author in a complex, emerging interdisciplinary field. The conscientious interdisciplinary research reflected in the text and footnotes of *The Patient as Person* thus became a model for all young scholars in the field.

There is a third characteristic of the Kennedy Institute that has also been present since the time of the Institute's inception—its *pluralism*, or, if the phrase does not sound too religious, its *ecumenical character*. I attribute this openness, this generosity of spirit, to both the Shrivers and André Hellegers. The pluralistic approach to intellectual inquiry also fit well with the ideals of Jesuit higher education, already visible in the early 1970s and, in my view, even more clearly embodied at Georgetown University today.

I can only speculate about how André Hellegers became such an open and tolerant leader and colleague. The Dutch Catholicism into which André was born in 1926 had a distinctive character. At that time the Catholic Church in the Netherlands had to coexist with several Protestant denominations, an influential Jewish community, and a culture that had been strongly influenced by secular humanism. In Britain, where he was educated by the Jesuits at Stonyhurst, André would have been under no illusions about Catholic domination of a culture or a legal system. That role at the time was played by the Church of England, although even its grip on the law was gradually slipping. In addition, both the Dutch and the British have been pioneers in the development of democratic theory and democratic institutions. We should also not forget the probable impact of Vatican II on the young André Hellegers. In major documents of the Council, Catholics were urged to rethink their earlier approaches to the other major Christian traditions and to non-Christian faiths, especially Judaism.

Sargent and Eunice Kennedy Shriver were raised in American Catholicism, in Baltimore and Boston, respectively. Through their active participation in public life at the local and national levels, they were well aware that people of good will from multiple religious traditions and from no religious tradition could work together for the benefit of the least well off, especially people with intellectual disabilities. Thus, it was no accident that the 1967 international conference on abortion included multiple viewpoints, even if conservative attendees outnumbered liberals. The film "Who Should Survive?"—about an infant with Down's syndrome who was not given lifesaving surgery—includes a panel discussion in which John Fletcher, then an Episcopal clergyman, urges his fellow panel members not to be too harshly critical of families who face agonizing decisions about the life or death of their newborn infants. The Shrivers also invited Robert G. Edwards to the October 1971 symposium, knowing full well that they would disagree with his position on human embryo research. Finally, we should not forget that Paul Ramsey was an ordained Methodist minister and theologian. On some issues Paul may have been slightly more Catholic than the Pope, but he was nonetheless a lifetime Protestant. Despite that fact, the Shrivers and André chose him to pioneer in the intensive study of ethical issues in medicine and biomedical research.

As a young Protestant joining the Kennedy Institute in 1971, I wondered how my work and my perspective on ethics would be received. Would non-Catholics be relegated to second-class status at the Kennedy Institute or at Georgetown University more generally? These worries were totally unfounded, as I encountered a warm and appreciative reception from André and an initial group of wonderful Catholic colleagues—Warren Reich, Charles Curran, and Richard McCormick. The ecumenism of the early 1970s extended quite easily to Protestants, and within the Kennedy Institute the circle of welcome was quickly extended to include Jewish colleagues and, later, Muslim colleagues, as well. Over the years our ranks have also included secular humanists and agnostics. Within this pluralism of viewpoints, there has always existed a most attentive and profound respect for our colleagues—often coupled with an active curiosity about the religious practices of faith communities whose traditions we do not know well.

How rich the pluralistic tradition at the Kennedy Institute has been can be illustrated with a few examples. In the 1970s the late John Connery did much of the research for his book on abortion in the Catholic theological tradition at the Kennedy Institute. For the past several years our colleague Margaret Little has been doing research for her two books on the morality of abortion. I think that it is fair to say that no one will confuse the positions for which these two scholars argue or the conclusions that they reach. Similarly, Tom Beauchamp and Edmund Pellegrino regularly debate the issue of voluntary assisted death. Neither has convinced the other on either the ethical or the public policy question, yet each faculty member continues to respect the other—and to engage in further dialogue. A striking example of this pluralism occurs so routinely in our Bioethics Library that we sometimes fail to notice it. In identifying and gathering materials for the library, our library and information science colleagues are scrupulous about collecting the best-documented and best-argued materials on any bioethical topic, without regard to the authors' viewpoints. This even-handed philosophy of collection development leads to a similar neutrality and objectivity in the work of our bibliographers and reference librarians. Every library patron can rest assured that the materials included in our databases or recommended to remote and local patrons will fairly represent all major viewpoints on a topic. Finally, Warren

Reich edited both the first and second editions of the *Encyclopedia of Bioethics* with meticulous attention to including a plurality of viewpoints on all topics covered.

I would also like to acknowledge the forbearance that Sargent and Eunice Kennedy Shriver have manifested toward the academic work of the Institute over the past thirty years. As you know, the relationships between donors and universities are not always wrinkle-free. I should also admit that there have been times when the Kennedy Foundation would have liked to see us do more research and writing on topics directly related to people with intellectual disabilities. At the same time, however, the Shrivers have displayed a keen understanding of the difference between public advocacy and careful scholarly work. A decisive moment in our relationship occurred in 1973. In the wake of *Roe v. Wade*, the issue of research on living fetuses became a major public policy issue. As I will explain in a moment, André Hellegers helped to ensure that the question of NIH support for such research became a matter of public record: the research was soon being discussed by the *Washington Post*, and a congressman from New York state proposed federal legislation that would have banned all research involving live human fetuses.

At this critical moment, André received a phone call from Eunice Kennedy Shriver asking us to take a position on fetal research as an Institute. I will never forget the discussion that our small band of faculty members held about how to respond to this important request. Our consensus was that no university or college or research institute should ever take a position on a specific public policy question *as an academic institution*. We did agree that several of us would study the issues surrounding fetal research as individual scholars, and that we would seek to make our possibly divergent conclusions known through a variety of channels. The Shrivers readily accepted this reply. As a result, a clear differentiation of function occurred. Maria Shriver led a group of concerned students from a local private school on a march to NIH, where the students demanded that NIH stop supporting live-fetus research. Some of us at the Institute wrote articles on the topic, and three of us later submitted testimony on fetal research to the National Commission for the Protection of Human Subjects. Perhaps aided by our testimony, the commission did in fact propose a middle way that protected pregnant women and living fetuses from invasive or damaging research, yet left the door open for minimal-risk studies that treated all fetuses equally.

A seminal work that exemplifies the Institute's ongoing commitment to pluralism is Tom Beauchamp and Jim Childress's *Principles of Biomedical*

Ethics. This book may seem a paradoxical choice because it has sometimes been subjected to criticism as a work that promotes a single point of view—the Georgetown mantra or principlism. A closer examination of the successive editions of the *Principles* reveals that such critiques are, at least in part, misguided. From the first edition forward, Tom and Jim have acknowledged a pluralism in their own approaches to ethical theory. In their words:

> For one author of this volume rule utilitarianism is preferable to any deontological theory presently available, while for the other, rule deontology is more acceptable than utilitarianism. (Beauchamp and Childress 1979, 40)

The authors go on to note that proponents of either theory may discover that they agree on the most important principles of ethics and in their judgments about particular cases.

Tom and Jim's pluralistic approach in *Principles of Biomedical Ethics* has also gone several steps further. The authors have refused to assign a higher priority to any one of their four principles over the other three—although it should be noted that (respect for) autonomy has always been discussed first. Thus, they acknowledge the potential relevance of any or all principles to any decision or policy. Further, Tom and Jim have always accepted an important role for virtue theory as a complementary mode of ethical analysis to their own approach, which focuses primarily on the principles and rules governing moral action. In fact, in the most recent edition of their work the discussion of virtue theory precedes the action-oriented discussion of principles. Finally, the Beauchamp-Childress list of alternative ethical theories has grown from edition to edition, so that in the most recent edition liberal individualism, communitarianism, and an ethics of care are treated as worthy rivals to utilitarianism and Kantianism (Beauchamp and Childress 2001, 355–77).

There is a wimpy kind of pluralism that simply does not care how sloppy people's arguments are or how irrational their conclusions may be. This is not the kind of pluralism that has characterized the work of the Kennedy Institute. I must therefore hasten to identify a fourth and final feature of our early history—*the courageous search for truth, no matter how difficult the search and no matter how painful or unpopular the truth turns out to be.*

For me, the most vivid illustration of this courage is to be found in an article written by André Hellegers in 1968 or early 1969, before the

Kennedy Institute was founded. André supported the majority recommendation of the Papal Commission on Birth Control, which would have liberalized the church's position on several modes of contraception. He was deeply disappointed by Pope Paul VI's rejection of the majority view in the 1968 encyclical *Humanae Vitae*. André's response to the encyclical in a 1969 book edited by Charles Curran was titled "A Scientist's Analysis." This short article is one of the most anguished and passionate essays that André ever wrote. It is still worth reading thirty-three years later.

In this seminal essay André Hellegers, a Catholic layman, asked a very simple yet profound question: What role, if any, can scientific information play in the church's attempts to formulate ethical guidance for its members? As a Protestant, I was amazed at the directness and forcefulness of André's dissent.

Two paragraphs from André's essay deserve to be quoted and pondered:

> For the scientist the encyclical presents a number of puzzling aspects: in the first place comes the absence of scientific evidence for, or indeed of scientific thought in reaching, the conclusions which the encyclical draws. Secondly, the scientist is struck by the absence of biological considerations in the entire encyclical. It is striking that the first section, which deals with "New Aspects," and which alludes to demographic, sociological, and educational problems, nowhere acknowledges that there might have been new biological facts of importance discovered since the encyclical *Casti Connubii* [1930]. . . . Equally interesting, but more ominous in this context, is paragraph 6. Here it is made clear that nothing that a present or future scientist could possibly contribute in terms of scientific data could have any pertinence to the subject, if certain criteria of solutions would emerge which departed from the moral teaching of marriage proposed with constant firmness by the teaching authority of the Church. To the scientist it is difficult to see why the Papal Commission should have been called at all. The teaching proposed with constant firmness by the Church was well known before the [c]ommission was appointed, and it did not require the energy and financial expenditures involved in bringing several dozen consultants to Rome to gather information if, *a priori*, such information was to be eliminated if it led to different conclusions than in the past.

The implications of this paragraph extend far beyond the subject of contraception. The wording of the paragraph is of cardinal importance for the relationship between science and theology. The paragraph implies that theology need not take into account scientific data, but shall reach its conclusions regardless of present or future facts. Had the encyclical stated that the data, advanced by the commission, were wrong or irrelevant, or were insufficient to warrant a change in teaching, that would have been one thing. It is quite another thing to imply that agreement with past conclusions is the *sine qua non* for acceptance of a study. Such wording pronounces the scientific method of inquiry irrelevant to Roman Catholic theology. (Hellegers 1969, 216–17)

From what sources did André derive such courage and such inner freedom? Again, we can only attempt to reconstruct some of the factors. (I wish that we could ask André to help us in the effort.) As Warren Reich has pointed out in an illuminating essay in the *Kennedy Institute of Ethics Journal*, André's parents had both been involved in resisting political oppression in Europe (Reich 1999, 33–34). His family escaped Belgium by boat literally minutes in advance of Hitler's invading armies. As a thirteen-year-old, André was an exile in a new land. Given this heritage and a brush with death as a teenager, André undoubtedly developed the capacity to distinguish between important and trivial issues. He would also have been keenly aware of Hitler's tyranny and the suffering that German expansionism had inflicted on his immediate and extended family, as well as on all of Europe. Thus, it would not be surprising if he had developed a wariness about the potential misuses of state power—and perhaps a certain skepticism about authority in general.

Warren Reich's thorough research on André's life and thought has uncovered that Belgian Cardinal Désiré Mercier was a role model for André during his entire lifetime (Reich 1999, 34). I am embarrassed to admit that I knew nothing about Cardinal Mercier before reading Warren's essay. A few hours of research with books borrowed from the Woodstock Library revealed why this brave Belgian would have captured André's imagination. First, Cardinal Mercier was a scholar, who helped to recapture but also to reform the Thomistic tradition in the late nineteenth century. Equally important, I am sure, was the Cardinal's passion for justice and his willingness to take risks in the midst of oppression. When the German armies invaded neutral Belgium in August 1914, at the beginning of World War I, they burned the venerable library of the University of Louvain, murdered at least forty Catholic priests, and shot to death literally hundreds of innocent civilians. In his pastoral letter to all the congregations of his diocese in December 1914, Cardinal Mercier decried the aggression and brutality of the German army, citing many of the murdered priests by name (Mercier 1917, 3–36; Boileau 1997, 383–93). Within days the German army sought to confiscate all copies of Mercier's pastoral letter and placed the Cardinal himself under house arrest. For the remainder of the war Cardinal Mercier was steadfast in denouncing German atrocities and in attempting to move the Vatican away from what the Cardinal considered a weak-kneed neutrality, as the Holy See attempted to maintain good relationships with both German and Belgian Catholics (Horne and Kramer 2001, 267–77). We are indebted to the research of Warren Reich for the insight that André Hellegers's mother also participated in the Belgian resistance to German occupation (Reich 1999, 33–34).

In André's own life and work, there are several striking examples of his courage and willingness to protect dissent. The first two Catholic theologians whom André invited to the Kennedy Institute were Warren Reich and Charles Curran. Both had been active in the attempt to reform Catholic moral theology in the late 1960s, and Warren Reich had been a visible and active supporter of Charles Curran when Catholic University and the Vatican had tried to set limits on the scope of his theological inquiries. Warren was the first long-term Catholic scholar at the Institute, and Charles Curran our first visiting scholar. In 1974 and 1975, André invited Bernard Häring, another burr under the Vatican's saddle, to join us as a visiting scholar. To André, who was supported by the Shrivers in all these decisions, inviting conscientious, controversial scholars to pursue their academic work at the Kennedy Institute was as natural as breathing.

The late Richard McCormick is another interesting case in point. Although he was considerably older than either Warren Reich or Charles Curran, he also periodically ran afoul of church authorities because of his innovative work in moral theology. I remember an illuminating conversation with Dick in the early 1980s in which I expressed concern that he was under investigation by church authorities in Rome because of statements contained in some of his writings. Dick replied, in his typical, self-deprecating manner, "LeRoy, I'm sort of a sacred cow in Catholic theology. Besides, I'm too old to be a prime target for a formal investigation." This was the man whom André and Georgetown University President Robert Henle, in consultation with the Shrivers, chose to be the first holder of the Rose F. Kennedy Chair in Christian Ethics in 1973. Between that year and the time of André's death in 1979, I am sure that there were many occasions on which André ran interference for Dick to protect the freedom of his academic work.

André also had little patience with government authorities who he thought were abusing their authority or misleading the public. As I mentioned earlier, the issue of research on living human fetuses became a matter of intense public debate in 1973. André was a key figure in starting that debate. NIH—and one spokesperson for NIH, in particular—had repeatedly assured the press and the public that NIH was not funding *any* live-fetus research. From his prior work on an NIH study section, André knew that the NIH spokesperson was lying. This kind of duplicity in answer to direct inquiries by the press drove André right up the proverbial wall. I will not venture to repeat some of the epithets that our incensed former director privately hurled at the NIH official. Suffice it to say, "meathead" would have been one of the milder terms that André used to characterize his adversary. How did the truth emerge about what NIH was actually doing? I can assert with confidence that André Hellegers did not directly deliver confidential documents to the press. However, I will admit that André left critical and incriminating evidence in a place where an enterprising reporter from *Ob-Gyn News* could readily find it. The truth about NIH's cover-up broke first in this throwaway newsletter, and within days the *Washington Post* had also picked up the story. From the *Post*, it was only a short step to Capitol Hill. Confronted by the evidence, NIH had no choice but to back down and to acknowledge its support of research on living fetuses.

The feisty spirit of a person like André Hellegers lives on long after the person himself has passed away. I would like to illustrate this enduring influence with a vignette from the work of our colleague Ruth Faden, who was at the Institute and worked with André only during the last three years of his life. Ruth was appointed chair of the Advisory Committee on Human Radiation Experiments in 1994. Two or three years ago, as I was talking with Ruth about her work with ACHRE, she recounted a story that I know André would have thoroughly enjoyed. According to Ruth, during her initial meetings with officials from the Clinton administration, she was told, "In your committee work, please stay away from three topics—the atomic veterans, the Marshall Islanders (from the vicinity of the nuclear tests), and the uranium miners. The U.S. government has dealt with the questions about these groups, and there is no need to dredge up these controversial topics again." My curiosity was piqued.

"So, what did you and your committee do, Ruth?" The answer came back immediately: "We studied all three groups and discussed them in our report." I was dumbfounded. "But, Ruth, you'd been warned not to study or discuss those topics. Didn't it require a bit of courage for you and the staff and the committee members to defy your instructions?" I will never forget Ruth's response: "So, LeRoy, what was the government going to do when we explored the forbidden topics—fire the whole committee?" André would have been delighted with this reply.

As I prepared this chapter, I thought of other major characteristics of the Kennedy Institute. For example, though we began as a research institute only, we gradually became involved in teaching at multiple levels, thanks in part to the gentle prodding of the Kennedy Foundation. I also reflected on the serendipity involved in our being physically located on a liberal-arts campus rather than in a medical center. In addition, I mused about how our location in Washington, D.C., made it almost inevitable that we would be drawn into discussing public policy questions, as well as more classical issues in moral philosophy and theology. Finally, I remembered the inscription below the bust of André Hellegers in the Bioethics Library, which urges us to "combine competence and compassion" in all that we attempt to do. However, these themes will have to wait for the Institute's *fortieth* anniversary celebration.

In summary, the four features of the Kennedy Institute that I have identified are its international focus, its interdisciplinary character, its pluralism, and the courage of its members in their search for truth. These characteristics are exemplified in the seminal works on bioethics that we have considered. Thanks to the vision and generosity of André Hellegers and the Shrivers, we who read these works can remember and celebrate both the beauty and the power of our heritage.

NOTE

1. This essay was later included in Paul's 1970 book *Fabricated Man* (Ramsey 1970b, 1–59).

REFERENCES

Beauchamp, Tom L., and James F. Childress. 1979. *Principles of Biomedical Ethics.* New York: Oxford University Press.

———. 2001. *Principles of Biomedical Ethics.* 5th ed. New York: Oxford University Press.

Boileau, David A. 1997. *Cardinal Mercier: A Memoir.* Leuven: Peeters.

Hellegers, André E. 1969. A Scientist's Analysis. In *Contraception: Authority and Dissent*, edited by Charles E. Curran. New York: Herder and Herder.

Horne, John, and Alan Kramer. 2001. *German Atrocities, 1914: A History of Denial*. New Haven, Conn.: Yale University Press.

Mercier, Désiré. 1917. *Cardinal Mercier: Pastorals, Letters, Allocutions, 1914–1917*. New York: P. J. Kenedy & Sons.

Ramsey, Paul. 1956. Freedom and Responsibility in Medicine and Sex Ethics: A Protestant View. *New York University Law Review* 31: 1189–1204.

————. 1966. Moral and Religious Implications of Genetic Control. In *Genetics and the Future of Man: A Discussion*, edited by John D. Roslansky. New York: Appleton-Century-Crofts: 107–69.

————. 1970a. *The Patient as Person: Explorations in Medical Ethics*. New Haven, Conn.: Yale University Press.

————. 1970b. *Fabricated Man: The Ethics of Genetic Control*. New Haven, Conn.: Yale University Press.

Reich, Warren T., ed. 1978. *Encyclopedia of Bioethics*. 4 vols. New York: Free Press.

————, ed. 1995. *Encyclopedia of Bioethics*. Revised ed. 5 vols. New York: Simon and Schuster Macmillan.

————. 1999. The "Wider View": André Hellegers's Passionate, Integrating Intellect and the Creation of Bioethics. *Kennedy Institute of Ethics Journal* 9: 25–51.

Walters, LeRoy, and Tamar Joy Kahn, eds. 2002. *Bibliography of Bioethics*. Volume 28. Washington, D.C.: Kennedy Institute of Ethics, Georgetown University.

CONTRIBUTORS

Tom L. Beauchamp, Ph.D., has a joint appointment as professor of philosophy in the Philosophy Department at Georgetown University and as a senior research scholar in the Kennedy Institute of Ethics.

Lisa Sowle Cahill, Ph.D., is the J. Donald Monan, S.J., Professor of Theology at Boston College. Her most recent book is *Family: A Christian Social Perspective* (Augsberg Fortress, 2000).

James F. Childress, Ph.D., is the John Allen Hollingsworth Professor of Ethics and Professor of Medical Education at the University of Virginia, where he directs the Institute for Practical Ethics. From 1975 to 1979, he was the Joseph P. Kennedy, Sr. Professor of Christian Ethics at the Kennedy Institute of Ethics at Georgetown University.

Charles E. Curran, S.T.D., is Elizabeth Scurlock University Professor of Human Values at Southern Methodist University. His latest book is *Catholic Social Teaching 1891–Present: A Historical, Theological, and Ethical Analysis* (Georgetown University Press, 2002).

H. Tristram Engelhardt, Jr., Ph.D., M.D., is professor in the Department of Philosophy at Rice University, and professor emeritus at Baylor College of Medicine. His most recent book is *The*

Foundations of Christian Bioethics (Swets and Zeitlinger, 2000).

Patricia A. King, J.D., is the Carmack Waterhouse Professor of Law, Medicine, Ethics, and Public Policy at Georgetown University Law Center and adjunct professor in the Department of Health Policy and Management, School of Hygiene and Public Health at Johns Hopkins University.

Eran P. Klein, Ph.D., is currently completing his M.D. at the Georgetown University School of Medicine.

William F. May, Ph.D., is the Cary M. Maguire University Professor of Ethics Emeritus at Southern Methodist University.

Edmund D. Pellegrino, M.D., is the Professor Emeritus of Medicine and Medical Ethics at the Center for Clinical Bioethics at Georgetown University Medical Center. He was the John Carroll Professor of Medicine and Medical Ethics and the former director of the Kennedy Institute of Ethics, the Center for the Advanced Study of Ethics at Georgetown University, and the Center for Clinical Bioethics.

Warren T. Reich, S.T.D., is Distinguished Research Professor of Religion and Ethics and Professor Emeritus of Bioethics at Georgetown University.

Robert M. Veatch, Ph.D., is professor of medical ethics at the Kennedy Institute of Ethics, Georgetown University. He also holds appointments as professor of philosophy and adjunct professor in the Department of Community and Family Medicine at Georgetown's Medical Center, and was a former director of the Kennedy Institute. He is the author of the second edition of *The Basics of Bioethics* (Prentice Hall, 2003).

Jennifer K. Walter is an M.D./Ph.D. student of philosophy at Georgetown University.

LeRoy Walters, Ph.D., is the Joseph P. Kennedy, Sr. Professor of Christian Ethics at the Kennedy Institute of Ethics, Georgetown University, and a professor of philosophy at Georgetown. He was one of the former directors of the Kennedy Institute of Ethics. In 2003 he coedited the sixth edition of *Contemporary Issues in Bioethics* with Tom L. Beauchamp (Wadsworth).

INDEX